THERAPEUTIC RECREATION INTERVENTION
An Ecological Perspective

THERAPEUTIC RECREATION INTERVENTION
An Ecological Perspective

Roxanne Howe-Murphy
San Jose State University

Becky G. Charboneau
U.S.–U.S.S.R. Youth Exchange Program

Prentice-Hall, Inc., Englewood Cliffs, New Jersey 07632

Library of Congress Cataloging-in-Publication Data

Howe-Murphy, Roxanne.
   Therapeutic recreation intervention.

   Includes bibliographies and index.
   1. Recreational therapy.   2. Handicapped—Services
for   3. Rehabilitation.   I. Charboneau, Becky G.
II. Title. [DNLM: 1. Handicapped.   2. Recreation.
3. Rehabilitation.   4. Social Environment.   QT 250 H8569t]
RM736.7.H69   1987   615.8'5153   86–25268
ISBN 0-13-914656-3

Editorial/production supervision
   and interior design: Virginia L. McCarthy
Cover design: 20/20 Services, Inc.
Manufacturing buyer: Harry P. Baisley

Prentice-Hall
Series in Leisure and Recreation
Joseph J. Bannon and James F. Murphy, Editors

Printed in the United States of America

10 9 8 7 6 5 4 3 2 1

ISBN 0-13-914656-3 01

Prentice-Hall International (UK) Limited, *London*
Prentice-Hall of Australia Pty. Limited, *Sydney*
Prentice-Hall Canada Inc., *Toronto*
Prentice-Hall Hispanoamericana, S.A., *Mexico*
Prentice-Hall of India Private Limited, *New Delhi*
Prentice-Hall of Japan, Inc., *Tokyo*
Prentice-Hall of Southeast Asia Pte. Ltd., *Singapore*
Editora Prentice-Hall do Brasil, Ltda., *Rio de Janeiro*

This book is dedicated to our parents:

Clayton and Grace Charboneau

and

Emily and Earl Howe

CONTENTS

PREFACE

This book represents another step in the evolution of recreation and leisure services for individuals with disabilities. As the professional practice of therapeutic recreation has evolved over the past several decades, two distinct models of intervention have emerged. The clinical or medical model focuses primarily on the individual. From this perspective, the individual possesses the deficits and is the target of change intervention. The social reform or community development model, on the other hand, perceives the environment as faulty. Thus, efforts are primarily directed at society as the focus of change. The ecological perspective of service delivery presented in this text integrates and expands these two models of intervention. From this perspective, change is seen as a process that naturally occurs as a result of the dynamic interaction between people and their environments. Within the process of intervention, this relationship is acknowledged and utilized. This perspective applies current concepts in the field of sociology and psychology to current practices in the field of therapeutic recreation. Discussions with professionals nationwide indicate that the ecological perspective is currently being practiced, it just has not been articulated in any systematic form in therapeutic recreation prior to this book.

The basic premise of this text rests on the recognition of the complex relationship between people and their environments. This approach focuses on the evolutionary and adaptive view of human beings, provides a framework for service delivery, and integrates intervention strategies for people and their environments. As we facilitate this development of individuals' adaptive capacities and improve the supportive qualities of their environments, mutual interdependence can be achieved and we thus begin to understand the nature of transformation. This premise not only provides a structure for analyzing concepts and transactions but also contributes to the development of the theory and practice of therapeutic recreation.

A profession is more than a set of practices, standards, and services. At the heart of any profession, organization, or institution are the people who deliver services to their constituencies. This in itself implies that as human beings we carry with us beliefs, values, perceptions, and attitudes regarding the individuals, communities, and professional organizations we serve. Today we are challenged to respond to the social and human evolution in our society and to assume an affirmative lead in human and health services. These challenges confront existing services, professional roles, and both professional and lay relationships. However, the primary challenge is directed toward each of us individually. Although we look to a profession for knowledge and direction, the ultimate responsibility rests with each of us.

This book, then, is primarily about *us*—as members of communities and organizations. It is about our attitudes, beliefs, and values, and it recognizes that the personal and professional judgments we make are based upon these determinants. Gerald S. Fain, Ph.D., an influential voice, colleague, and friend, has often reminded us that our decisions and consequent actions have the potential to be either helpful or harmful to others. As therapeutic recreation professionals we have the potential to be effective agents of change within agencies, organizations, medical institutions, and the community at large. As we become sensitive to the messages that we convey through practices and through language, we can have the power to influence policies and people. It is the authors' hope that this text will assist students and professionals in understanding themselves and their influence on the environments to ensure that recreation and play opportunities contribute to the quality of life for all individuals.

The primary focus of this book is the therapeutic recreation process, and this process can apply to all people. We live in a rapidly changing age in which people are confronted with stresses in every part of their lives. Generic leisure service professionals have a responsibility to assist all members of their community to become more leisure able. Often this involves much more than the management of resources, such as facilities and staff. The therapeutic recreation intervention process is one that can be used to assist people to cope and adapt to their environments and effect change in their lives. In addition, this perspective is viable because people with disabilities or illnesses are being forced to return to the community more rapidly because of new legislation that sets the number of days that facilities will be reimbursed for the care given to those in their charge. Community-based professionals must be more prepared to deal with a more diverse population than has been true in the past.

This book reflects the authors' own research and professional practice in segregated, therapeutic, and integrated environments working with both nondisabled and disabled persons. It also stems from hours of discourse with other colleagues, consumers, parents, and allied health and human service professionals. The text is the result of a coordinated attempt over the last several years to develop materials and resources that could be used in both university and organizational settings.

As an introductory work, this book has application in a variety of courses, and it is directed at students preparing to work both in specialized therapeutic settings (for example, hospitals, clinics, schools) and community settings (youth clubs, municipal recreation departments, commercial settings, environmental education programs, and so forth). While it is intended specifically for use in introductory therapeutic recreation courses, it will also be useful in mainstreaming courses. It is hoped that this text will provide both a helpful mechanism for integrating therapeutic and nontherapeutic option students into courses to facilitate a necessary exchange of ideas and to assist students in therapeutic recreation to develop a better understanding of their role in society.

Over the past fifteen years the authors have grown together as professional colleagues and personal friends. This time span represents many of the most meaningful moments together in this profession. The field of leisure has a special place in our hearts, and it is with an awareness of current practices and philosophy, coupled with our concern for the future direction of our world as a whole, that we desire to share these concerns by presenting an alternative way of looking at both our profession and life in general. This book reflects a vision we have seen together.

A SPECIAL RECOGNITION

Without Dr. James F. Murphy, this book would not have happened. Jim, partner, dearly loved friend, colleague, teacher and mentor, believed in our ability to produce a text which would provide another way of understanding this complex field. It was his undying faith and his assistance with the early developmental and conceptual phases of the manuscript that propelled us to undertake this task. Jim, with full hearts, we thank you.

ACKNOWLEDGMENTS

There are many individuals who have been extremely helpful to us during the development of this manuscript. Raymond O'Connell, our first editor, has been a vigilant friend and colleague throughout the development of this work. Ray's belief in us, and his occasional prodding, always intertwined with lots of humor is gratefully appreciated and acknowledged.

Several of our colleagues have served as reviewers throughout the development of this work. Some remain anonymous to us, but their comments have been most helpful in the subsequent revisions. To Dr. Peter A. Witt and Kathy Collard, a special thank you for their very valuable assistance.

Thanks to Dr. Paul Brown, Chair in the Department of Recreation and Leisure Studies at San Jose State University for his encouragement. And to John Williams, Director of Sunnyvale Parks and Recreation Department, who taught us the value of merging theory and practice, our sincere appreciation. Special thanks to Daisy Joseph who stood by us in typing and retyping portions of the manuscript, and to the many students in the Introduction to Therapeutic Recreation classes at San Jose State University, who offered suggestions in the early drafts of this work.

We would also like to extend a thank you to all those at Prentice-Hall who have assisted us in the preparation of the manuscript, particularly Emily Baker, Joseph Heider, and Virginia McCarthy.

This type of work does not get completed without the support of close colleagues, friends, and family. To these people: Don Bauer, Sam Bozzo, Gay Carpenter, Clay and Diana Charboneau, Kathy Halberg, Annie Head, Cheri Huber, Anne Idema, Randy Klein, Bill Michaelis, Suzanne Mirviss, Erin Murphy, the Murphy Family, Ann Nathan, Jan Neri, the Ogden Family, Mae Stadler, thank you for tolerating our moments of insanity with your love.

And finally, we cannot go without acknowledging the organization and its people who provided the environment in which our perspective about the field had its beginnings. To Richard Sandberg, Executive Director of United Cerebral Palsy Association of San Diego County and to Terri Spahr, who challenged us to grow, goes our deep appreciation.

Roxanne Howe-Murphy
San Jose State University
San Jose, California

Becky Charboneau
U.S.–U.S.S.R. *Youth Exchange Program*
San Francisco, California

AN INTRODUCTION TO THERAPEUTIC RECREATION
An Ecological Perspective of Service Delivery

An elderly man who is a new resident of a convalescent home initially spends much of his time sitting alone in his room listening to the radio. Encouraged by the therapeutic recreator, he gradually begins to volunteer information on his life's activities. After several weeks, the discovery that the man directed his church choir for several years leads to the formation of a new singing group in the home. The new resident is the group's director.

A 28-year-old woman prepares for her return to the community after three months' rehabilitation following an automobile accident. With the guidance and support of the therapeutic recreator at the rehabilitation center, she learns methods of adapting her favorite recreation activities so she can reinitiate her participation. Together, they also visit various community settings, such as concert facilities, theaters, and restaurants to identify accessible buildings and to learn strategies that will allow her to cope with people's reactions.

The recreation staff of both the Easter Seal Society and the YMCA in a small city work together to design and offer programs to mutually benefit participants allied with each agency. While all of the services provided through the YMCA are open and accessible to persons with disabilities, specific courses such as "Self-Defense and Fitness" are designed specifically to bring able-bodied and disabled individuals together.

A 14-year-old boy with a severe illness has been in a pediatric hospital for three weeks. It is projected that his stay will be extended for three or four more weeks for tests and treatment. After a staff meeting with the unit's doctors, nurses, social worker and allied therapists, the recreation therapist engages the young patient in a competitive board game at his bedside. During the game, the two talk informally and the boy begins to express his anguish over his confinement.

INTRODUCTION TO THE BOOK

The foregoing examples depict persons and situations with which therapeutic recreators are concerned.

> What elements do these scenarios have in common?
> In what ways is recreation important to the lives of individuals identified here?
> What relationship does therapeutic recreation have to each of these situations?

Herein begins the study of therapeutic recreation services. Based upon the limited sketches provided above, the reader would be correct in surmising that this examination encompasses a broad scope of material, including:

1. a range in the characteristics of persons served;
2. diverse purposes and functions of leisure services;
3. multiple types of environments in which services occur;
4. diverse professional roles, tools, and methods used to facilitate the change process.

Students and professionals alike find the scope encompassed in this area of study to be exciting and demanding, both in concept and in practice. The diversity is a result of many variables including the complexity of the society in which we live; the limitlessness of human endeavors; the varied personal and professional philosophies and orientations of service providers; and the range of interests, skills, and backgrounds that people attracted to this field bring with them. The diversity existing in concepts and manifested in practice is a mark of a discipline that is maturing in a rapidly evolving society. Because economic, technological, and social patterns in our society impact greatly upon the status of persons with disabilities, therapeutic recreation personnel are challenged to be at once analytical and responsive.

It is the intent of this book to present material and ideas in a conceptually logical framework and in the context of legal mandates and contemporary trends and issues, such as the demand for accountability and mainstreaming. An invitation is extended to each reader to explore this challenging field with an open mind and a bundle of curiosity.

It is the authors' hope that the material will be conceptually provocative and will provide a foundation for meaningful professional practice. We desire to raise new questions and provide some insights to long-raised concerns.

FACTORS CONTRIBUTING TO INTEREST IN, COMMITMENT TO, AND SERVICES FOR PERSONS WITH DISABILITIES

The values of recreation and leisure have long been espoused by advocates, and the interest in responsive services for persons with disabilities and illnesses has grown remarkably over the last few decades. The following discussion examines some possible reasons for this interest.

Societal factors.   Wars, because of the large number of wounded who return home, have often served to increase the visibility of disabled persons in society. Other factors in recent times have also contributed to a new awareness of disabled individuals. In the civil rights activities of the 1960s and 1970s, people with disabilities emerged with a more distinct profile in both the United States and Canada than had been true earlier. National and international efforts, such as the International Year of Disabled Persons in 1981, further highlighted the rights, abilities, interests, and activities of these people. Films, books, and other forms of media disseminated information on disabilities, environmental accessibility, and public attitudes. Advocates of the rights of disabled persons helped to bring about visible changes in the environment. The International Accessibility symbol (Figure 1-1) identified environments that permitted wheelchair users entrance and mobility within a building. Moreover, technological progress made possible devices that enable disabled individuals to participate in employment, education, recreation, and related endeavors in the mainstream of society. The use of braille, flashing lights, and beeping tones at crosswalks and in elevators and the use of sign language at forums and on television not only provide a means of communication to users, but also communicate to the public that individuals with disabilities are vital members of the community.

Legal factors.   Beginning in the late 1960s, several major pieces of federal legislation, such as the Education for All Handicapped Children Law and the Rehabilitation Act, were passed to protect the rights of persons with disabilities. Public agencies and settings receiving federal money were mandated to be accessible and to provide appropriate services. Litigation was used as a tool to gain and maintain basic human rights, including the rights to treatment, education, and protection from harm. These legal activities not

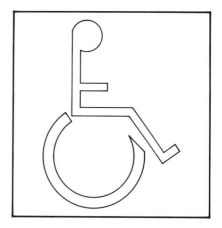

FIGURE 1-1 International Accessibility Symbol

only served to raise the awareness of the public but also benefitted able-bodied and disabled citizens.

Personal factors.   While the many social and legal activities raised the public consciousness about people with disabilities, more and more individuals were personally affected by disability. Medical advances in the last half of the twentieth century extended the longevity of those who decades earlier could not have survived severe impairments. Relatives, colleagues, social peers, and individuals themselves incurred and sustained the effects of illness and injury. Thus, more people came to understand personally the meaning of being disabled in a technological society. The importance of responsive and quality services and equal opportunities for all assumed greater meaning and consequence.

CONCEPTUAL FOUNDATIONS OF THERAPEUTIC RECREATION

Three conceptual areas serve to structure our understanding of therapeutic recreation. These areas provide foundations that help us to identify the commonalities that exist among therapeutic recreation services, regardless of the setting in which those services occur.

Foundation I: The Phenomena of Play, Recreation, and Leisure

Recreation, leisure, and play have assumed a critical place in the fabric of American life. In 1981, *U.S. News and World Report* magazine stated that economic expenditures for leisure pursuits exceeded those for national defense: $244 billion and $77 billion, respectively.[1] While nonfinancial expenditures are more difficult to quantify, there is ample evidence that recreation and leisure are considered crucial to the quality of life for many people.

"Life quality" is a rather nebulous term with profound implications. Personal definitions of this abstraction will vary for each of us, yet a commonality that undoubtedly would be reflected in most individual interpretations is the characteristic of excellence in our personal existence. Certainly this basic human issue is central to the questions raised by philosophers and scholars throughout history. To those seriously studying the impact of play, recreation, and leisure upon human existence, life quality serves as a focal issue.

Play, recreation, and leisure, though interrelated concepts, have each been studied extensively. Volumes have been written on the meaning of each concept. For the purposes of this book, leisure is defined as a state of mind. The individual defines what is and is not leisure. As such, leisure can occur at any time. This concept of leisure has been widely articulated.[2] Recreation refers to a freely chosen experience or an activity that often occurs during leisure. The activity leaves the participant feeling renewed and invigorated.

One approach to understanding play is to understand "playfulness." That is, rather than a specific activity (play) occurring under specific conditions, the style of participation (playfulness) is emphasized.[3] It has been suggested that the qualities of humor, manifest joy, and spontaneity are among those that characterize a playful style.[4] The importance of play to the human being has been well documented in the fields of leisure, psychology, and sociology. Play has been demonstrated to have inherent relationships to social, physical, and cognitive development;[5] to personality development needs;[6] to arousal needs and to a variety of human development concerns.[7]

Leisure is an area of our lives that provides pathways potentially leading to the attainment of desired excellence in our existence as human beings: personal fulfillment and dignity; control over our lives and independence; self-expression and inner joy. This state of being is sometimes referred to as *high-level wellness*.[8] In contemporary living, decisions are continually made which impact upon our lives. Throughout our life span, these decisions are, for the most part, determined by entities external to our personal existence. As children, our parents, teachers, and even older siblings assumed much of the responsibility for decision making. As we mature, we find decisions are imposed by employers, the government, and society as a whole. Thus, the amount of our individual freedom is restricted. Yet the areas in which we have personal control are, in many ways, central to our own self-identification and self-expression. Leisure potentially provides this freedom in our lives, as we choose to express ourselves in certain ways, choose to interact within certain environments and within selected social groupings. Through this self-determination, we have the possibility of discovering ourselves and satisfying our needs for dignity and self-esteem.

Playful, recreative, and leisurely experiences are defined individually. What one person finds fulfilling, another may find tedious. Play, recreation, and leisure potentially can occur in nearly any setting, alone or with others and within any time frame. It is apparent that these components of living cannot be extracted or isolated from other aspects of life. They are intricately intertwined with other forms of expression, with other life needs and interests. As such, they contribute to one's overall lifestyle.

To realize this type of experience, however, the appropriate conditions must exist, because play, recreation, and leisure are not automatic. For example, the individual must possess adequate information, skills, and resources, be they internal or external; and the person must possess an open attitude that allows for self-expression. A deficit in physical, cognitive, social, or emotional skills or resources necessary for certain experiences would undoubtedly result in excessive frustration or failure if the activity were undertaken.

Equally important, conditions must exist within the environment that encourage and allow play to be manifested. Variables, such as physical design, aesthetics, attitudes of others, and social networks play a major role in the degree to which personal satisfaction will occur. Thus, a deficient environment will frustrate or completely immobilize attempts to engage in meaningful experiences.

Leisure and its overall relationship to well-being provides the meaning behind therapeutic recreation service delivery. Without it, there is no reason for therapeutic recreation services. The relationship of leisure and various models of service delivery to persons with illness and disabilities are addressed in Chapter 3.

Foundation II: Ideology Toward Persons with Disabilities in Society

A second conceptual basis for leisure service provision is embodied in the ideology toward persons with disabilities in society. It is estimated that between 12 percent and 20 percent of people living in the United States, or between 36 million and 44 million people, have some type of physical, mental, or emotional disability.[9] The history of these individuals is not one of which society can be proud. Because of myths, fears, stereotypes, and ignorance, disabled persons in North America have a history of being consistently devalued. In the past, the manifestations of this devaluation have existed in every aspect of life. Limitations imposed upon disabled persons by society have taken an immense toll on personal freedom and lifestyle considerations, which, in turn, has often been reflected in unsatisfactory social relationships and networks, economic insecurity, and inadequate options in housing, transportation, education, and recreation.

Despite the progress cited earlier, there are numerous indications that the negative perceptions toward disabled persons really have not changed all that much. The use of very subtle cues—for example, quotes around the word *normal* (the disabled and the "normal")—points to an underlying belief that disabled persons are not normal or able. The message is that their ability does not really exist or, at most, has little significance to the rest of society. It is no wonder that people have contradictory feelings or perceptions about individuals with disabilities. The message is mixed: Yes, disabled persons exist and have rights; however, they are still very different from the rest of society and different does not equate with *good*. This perception may result in a lopsided and narrow perspective of such persons as "recipients" of services, who naturally assume the client/patient/helpee role. Despite the growing public awareness, the media have continued to present an image of the disabled "victim" who remains dependent. Opportunities for self-definition through a wide range of career, educational, recreational, and social experiences remain limited because of this restricted role definition.

come. The focus of this description is on the nature of the experience; the focus of change is the individual.

The National Therapeutic Recreation Society (NTRS), a national organization representing the profession, adopted a definition of therapeutic recreation that inclusively referred to a broad scope of services for persons with disabilities and illnesses, regardless of the setting in which services occurred. According to this definition, the purpose of therapeutic recreation is to "facilitate the development, maintenance, and expression of an appropriate leisure lifestyle" of these individuals.[12] Within this definition, therapeutic recreation encompasses services that utilize: (1) recreation activities as a means of therapy, (2) educational and counseling activities in developing self-awareness and leisure skills and resources, and (3) freely chosen recreational experiences to elicit pure, joyful play.[13]

Some writers in the field have found that definition overly broad. David Austin (1982) argued, "I object to the suggestion that a *primary* (his italics) role of therapeutic recreation specialists is that of a 'recreator for special populations' " (Gunn and Peterson, 1978, p. 23). He instead proposed that this is the role of community recreation personnel. He continued, "If there is a need to intervene with a special recreation program because certain special population group members are not willing or able to enter into self-directed leisure pursuit, the therapeutic recreation specialist should be responsible for the program."[14]

In a more recent text, Carter, Van Andel, and Robb also agreed that therapeutic recreation is an intervention-oriented process. They posited, "Therapeutic recreation may be viewed as a process or systematic use of recreation activities and experiences to achieve specific objectives. This process is not limited to certain categories of individuals or a particular setting. Rather, therapeutic recreation may be applicable to any individual whose needs and goals would seem to benefit from such an intervention."[15]

The American Therapeutic Recreation Association (ATRA), created in 1984 to represent a more specific aspect of the profession, stated that the "primary purpose of service is to promote the development of functional independence . . . primarily delivered, structured and administered in health care and human service settings with an emphasis on treatment and education of the clients served."[16] This definition also refers to a process of intervention, but one geared more toward clinical environments. The focus of change is primarily on the individual.

The use of the term *therapeutic recreation* throughout this text represents a continuing evolution of thought in the field. It is based on a recognition of the many elements necessary for play, and on a realization that functional impairments (disabling conditions) can be possessed by both the individual and the environment. Therefore, the term will refer to a planned process of intervention directed toward specific environmental and/or individual change. The goals of the change process are to maximize the quality of life, enhance the leisure functioning of the individual, and promote acceptance of persons with disabilities within the community. The processes by which purposeful change occurs are variable, encompassing both the promotion of abilities (individual, community, environment) and the elimination of individual and environmental barriers. This is known as the *ecological perspective.*

THE ECOLOGICAL PERSPECTIVE

> No man is an island entire of itself; every man is a piece of the continent, a part of the main. If a clod be washed away by the sea, Europe is the less, as well as if a promontory were, as well as if a manor of thy friend's or of thine own were. Any man's death diminishes me, because I am involved in mankind, and therefore never send to know for whom the bell tolls; it tolls for thee.
>
> John Donne, XVII Meditation

The interdependence of human beings upon one another and the mutual influence of individuals and their environments, the message so well captured by John Donne, form a central theme of this book. Some cultures have recognized and highly valued the relationship between individuals and their environments. The American Indians and Far Eastern philosophers are among those who have long expounded the intricate relationship of a unit to its parts, implying wholeness of any phenomenon.

Interdependence

Let us examine this concept of interdependence in the following case study.

> Wendy is a 14-year-old girl who lives with her mother, two older brothers, two dogs, three cats, and innumerable fish in a small town. Wendy's father left the family when Wendy was four. Wendy and her brothers attend the same junior-senior high school, where Wendy is doing well in the eighth grade. She is totally dependent physically. She has an attendant at school and uses adaptive equipment to help her be as independent as possible in other aspects of her life. For example, because she has very little control over her flailing arms and legs, she has a motorized wheelchair, which propels her forward, sideways, and backward with the touch of a joystick. Because she is nonverbal, her electronically controlled communication board enables her to express herself either on a screen for all to see or on a tickertape for more one-on-one or small-group conversation. Wendy enjoys school, being with her friends, and participating with her outdoor-loving family in diverse activities. Her frustration is apparent when she is confronted by architectural barriers that prevent her from moving freely into different settings.

If we analyze this situation, examining all the parts that make up the whole, we will discover the following:

A. About Wendy

EXAMPLES OF WHAT WE KNOW

- Wendy is successful in 8th grade, which is typical grade level for a 14-year-old.
- Wendy is nonverbal; has little control of limbs. She needs assistance with many personal hygiene tasks, but is relatively independent in a chair.
- Wendy enjoys interacting with family and friends.

EXAMPLES OF MISSING INFORMATION

- How does Wendy cope with frustrations caused by environmental barriers?
- What is Wendy's level of confidence and self-esteem?

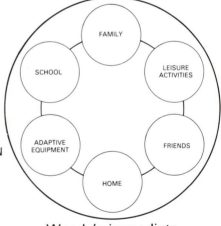

Wendy the person

B. About Wendy's Immediate Environment

EXAMPLES OF WHAT WE KNOW

- Electronic devices enable Wendy to communicate and move around.
- A regular junior-senior school admitted Wendy as a student.
- Wendy has a social (peer) network.
- Wendy's family apparently involves her in family activities.

EXAMPLES OF MISSING INFORMATION

- Does Wendy or the rest of the family have contact with the father?
- Does Wendy have friends of all ages, both sexes, disabled and able-bodied?
- What environments are inaccessible to Wendy?
- How is the expensive adaptive equipment paid for?

Wendy's immediate environment

FIGURE 1-2 A System Analysis

It is not difficult to begin imagining the impact of Wendy on her immediate environment, and of the environment on Wendy. It is obvious that if Wendy could not avail herself of an electric wheelchair or communication board, she would be much less independent. If she was more dependent, her family and friends would be directly affected. Perhaps Wendy would be forced to attend a different school, which could result in transportation problems and interfere with social interactions. This analysis provides a brief sketch of some of the factors that require recognition if we are to understand the complexity of any unit.

Understanding the "wholeness" of any situation requires effort, and often a rejection of the perspective with which people are well acquainted: namely, segmented or fragmented thinking. Certainly students who have reached the point where they are reading this text have experienced the fundamental fragmentation: education. To make teaching and learning easier, subjects are generally arbitrarily categorized into selected courses. Our life experience, however, reminds us that subjects or issues are not nearly so neatly classified in life as they are in education. A result of fragmentation is the separation of individuals from their environments. The Puritan Ethic, which emphasized individual strength and character in the face of all obstacles, is largely responsible for our preoccupation with "individual deficit" or "blaming the victim"[17] for his or her plight. For example, children who have a difficult time in school are often thought of as "unable." As a result, they are blamed for their failure to achieve academically, rather than looking to the educator to determine if there is a problem in the teaching style or level of materials being used. Education, social services, leisure services, medicine, psychology, and all forms of human services have found it most convenient to diagnose and treat the individual in isolation of the whole. Equally as fragmenting, many buildings have been constructed, many institutions designed, and many laws passed without any thought given to the relationship between these creations and the individuals whom they are intended to serve. Focusing on parts without taking into account the whole is archaic.

SOCIAL SYSTEMS THEORY

The ecological perspective is based upon the concept of systems, which provides a model for analyzing the relationship of interrelated and interdependent parts comprising a whole. *System* has been defined as

> a complex of elements or components directly or indirectly related in a causal network, such that each component is related to at least some others in a more or less stable way within a particular period of time.[18]

The social systems that are the focus of this book are composed of the interaction and influence among persons within their social, physical, aesthetic, and functional environments.[19] This perspective recognizes the complexity and intricacy of relationships among growing, developing individuals and changing environments.

Selected Characteristics of Social Systems

The following section briefly introduces selected characteristics of social systems that relate to the study of therapeutic recreation. *Organization* is a major characteristic of social systems. This concept refers to the identification, arrangement, and interdependencies of parts (referred to as "components") that comprise a whole (referred to as a "system"). This organization can be examined through use of a schematic drawing representing a system. For example, a total person as a system can be represented through a diagram identifying the primary components and their influence upon one another. Figure 1–3 suggests that if we are to understand an individual, we must consider all aspects of that person.

Holons, or levels of systems.   Any of the components depicted in Figure 1–3 can also be viewed as a system in its own right, consisting of various interdependent components. The concept that each component is simultaneously a part of a whole and a whole in its own right reflects another characteristic of a system, which is called a *holon*. This phenomenon was recognized in the Roman god Janus, who faces two directions at once—inward toward its own parts and outward to the system of which it is a part.[20] An understanding of the holon concept is critical in designating the "focal system" or the *primary* system of attention for the purposes of understanding and service delivery. For example, individual-oriented treatment typically des-

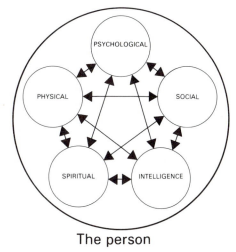

FIGURE 1–3 The Whole Person   The person

ignates the "person" as the focal system, or the focus of treatment. Social change typically identifies the "community" as the target of intervention. On the other hand, there has recently been much more focus on the importance of recognizing the family as part of the focus of intervention when an individual family member is manifesting problem behavior. Similarly, if an individual's leisure behavior is our primary concern, we must consider not only that person's inner characteristics (physical, social, mental, psychological status) but also recognize that the individual is part of a family, a peer network, and a community (see Figure 1–4).

Boundaries. Every component of a system is a part of other systems. Similarly, systems are a part of multiple suprasystems. Defining the boundaries or the limits of the system is essential in order to design and implement an intervention strategy that will impact upon an area of need.

Refer again to our friend Wendy. Let us say that her mother called the community's recreation department to inquire about enrolling Wendy in some of its programs. How much of Wendy's environment and of Wendy as an individual should be taken into account in involving her in programs of the department? In other words, what should be the boundaries of the service personnel's concerns?

Energy. Within every system there is a constant transfer of energy among parts of the system, as well as an exchange of energy between the system and the systems of which it is a part (called *suprasystem*). This flow of energy stresses the dynamic nature of systems. Resources and information give form to the energy and provide the system with the capacity to effect change. The energy exchanged within a system takes the form of *input, process, output,* and *feedback.*

> INPUT is the raw information and resources that are fed into a system.
> PROCESS is what happens among those elements (resources, information) when they interact within the system.
> OUTPUT is the result of the interaction or the outcome of the process.
> FEEDBACK is that information that is put back into the suprasystem, which can lead to a modification within the system.

For example, in Figure 1–5, the family contributes (provides input) established patterns of interaction, standards or levels of expectations, sources of

---

FIGURE 1–4   Systems and Their Boundaries. Adapted from Naomi Brill, *Working with People: The Helping Process* [Philadelphia, Pa.: J. B. Lippincott, 1973], p. 64.

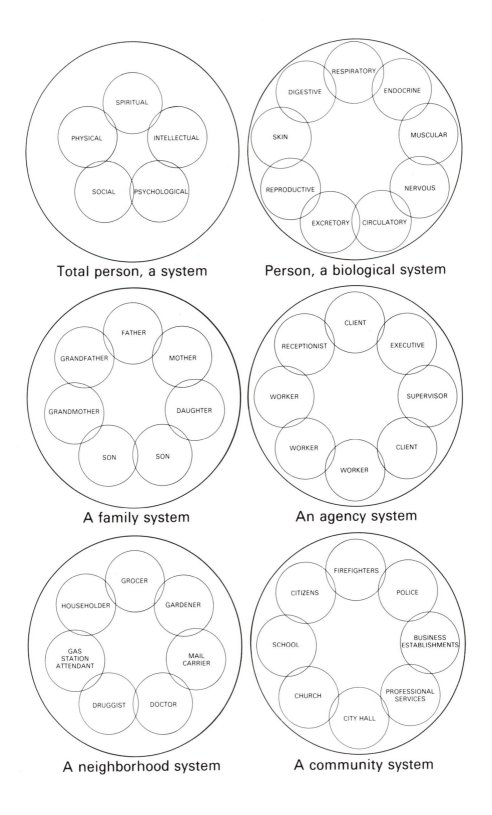

Total person, a system

Person, a biological system

A family system

An agency system

A neighborhood system

A community system

INPUT	PROCESS	OUTPUT
family members	interactions among members;	healthy family or
responsibilities	needs are/are not met by family;	family in-distress
behaviors	individual response to other member's	
resources	needs, behaviors	
expectations		

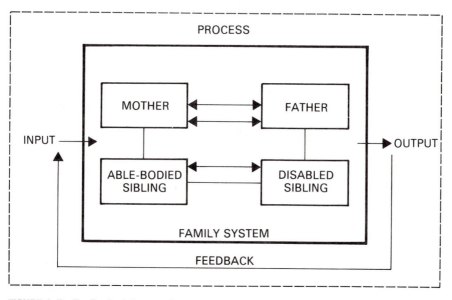

FIGURE 1-5 The Family: A Systems Perspective

physical maintenance (food, shelter), and security to the child. The child with a disability will also contribute selected behaviors and needs. The interaction of the family members, including the disabled child, comprises the process of this particular system. A child with disruptive behaviors may interrupt routine behaviors of the parents and siblings. The output of this system may well be a family in distress. The distress is fed back into the input (for example, expectations; routine behaviors in work and play of other family members). The family may adjust its expectations or interactions to better support the child. At any point in this input-process-output, the system may break down. For the family, this could result in increased frustration, quarreling, or even separation of family members from one another through divorce or out-of-home placement for the child. Given a different set of circumstances, this same family system could also flourish.

Let us take another example of a system undergoing change. During the early 1970s, many municipal and other publicly supported recreation and leisure service departments grew: Staff was added, programs were created, supplies and equipment could be purchased without a great deal of difficulty. In the mid-1970s something called the "taxpayer's revolt" took hold of the country. California was one of the first states to experience this phenomenon when voters approved Proposition 13, which severely limited the money going into the public coffers. With input (money, support for tax-dependent services) curtailed, these departments faced severe cutbacks in the form of personnel, facilities, and services. Departments formed liaisons with other public and private agencies, called upon volunteers, and urged community members to assume increased responsibilities for planning and conducting services. This is a clear example of how the suprasystem (the larger society) caused changes within the operations of the system (recreation and leisure service departments).

These examples demonstrate that this feedback may lead to adaptation: (1) within the system (the family), (2) between subsystems or systems (for example, recreation departments in communities), or (3) between the system and suprasystem. This is not a difficult concept to understand, but it is important. Let us look at another example to ensure that we are thinking along the same line. Recall our discussion about national, state, and local efforts to increase the ability of persons with disabilities to participate in the mainstream of society. Before the early 1960s, few laws protected the rights of this group of people. However, once people with disabilities became aware of their rights, they demanded that society address their concerns. Congress responded and passed a limited amount of legislation. Then, as legislation increased the access of disabled people to different aspects of society, the media began to present information to the public on the activities of various disabled persons. Slowly the public awoke to this segment of society. Disabled persons became more visible members of the community. Seen from a systems perspective, the legislative system received input from the larger social suprasystem, particularly from disabled consumers; it processed the information and passed laws (process) and provided output in the form of laws to the suprasystem.

THE APPLICATION OF SOCIAL SYSTEMS TO THERAPEUTIC RECREATION

The use of a social systems approach has many benefits for therapeutic recreators, as well as for other leisure service personnel. The following list is adapted from Brill in *Working with People: The Helping Process.*[21]

1. As an analytical tool, it assures that a unified perspective is utilized. It assists in assessing relationships, targeting important points of interaction, and anticipating results based upon a working knowledge of behavior.

2. As a tool for designating approaches to intervention, it takes the onus off the individual. In recreation, it recognizes those forces which influence the individual and identifies ways in which the individual impacts upon the environment.

3. It affects the role of the leisure services worker/therapeutic recreator by recognizing that the professional is a part of the system. Rather than serving in a central role, which attempts to enact a given intervention, the worker can assume an enabler role to facilitate change either on the part of the individual or within the environment. "This coincides with the basic principle that fundamental change comes from within the individual or system; it cannot be imposed. . . . "[22]

A social systems approach helps answer such questions as:

What is the focal system with which I should be concerned?
What are the boundaries of this system?
What are the "rules" governing these behaviors?
At what point does there appear to be a breakdown in the system?[23]

The worker can target problematic areas and work with the appropriate individuals within the system in designing an effective strategy for change. The professional's role may vary from providing direct services in the form of therapy or leisure education to providing community education, advocacy, or assisting individuals in accessing community resources.

In a book titled *Leisure Service Delivery System: A Modern Perspective,* the concept of systems in this field was introduced as "the interrelationships among people in their physical and social environment, and the way these relationships influence or are influenced by particular social processes."[24] The authors identified: (1) the participants, (2) the social environment, (3) the physical environment, and (4) leisure service organizations as critical components of the leisure service delivery system.[25] Murphy and Howard further characterized these four components in a later text.[26] See Table 1-1.

HUMAN ECOLOGY: AN APPLICATION OF THE SYSTEMS MODEL

The reader will note that Murphy and Howard use the term *ecology* in their conceptualization (see Table 1-1). Based on the social systems theory, the concept of human ecology "rests on the evolutionary, adaptive view of human beings in continuous transactions within the environment."[27] As a concept that recognizes the dynamic relationship between people and their environments, it can be utilized within all aspects of therapeutic recreation in addition to other services.

TABLE 1-1 Components [Ecology Design] of the Leisure Service Delivery System

SOCIAL COMPONENTS	PHYSICAL COMPONENTS	PARTICIPANT COMPONENTS	AGENCY COMPONENTS
Ethnicity	Climate	Human needs	Goals
Cultural heritage	Transportation	Motivation	Objectives
Social class	system	Individual self-	Philosophy
Race	Topography	concept	Organizational
Family	Business and	Age	structure
Mores/folkways	industry	Sex	Leadership
Religion	Schools	Experience	Recreation areas
Sanitation	Churches	Attitudes	and facilities
Education	Environmental	Interests	Open space
Allied humor	quality	Desires	Locality
Service resources	Population density/	Goals	Priorities
Justice/courts	crowdedness	Competencies	Financial support
		Capabilities	and distribution
			Equipment

James F. Murphy and Dennis R. Howard, *Delivery of Community Leisure Services: An Holistic Approach* (Philadelphia, PA.: Lea & Febiger, 1977) p. 121.

Application

The ecological perspective is useful in integrating two previously opposed positions of intervention in therapeutic recreation. The clinical or medical model focuses primarily on the individual. From this perspective, the individual possesses the deficits and is the target of change interventions. The social reform or community development model, favored by a smaller segment of the profession, perceives the environment as faulty. Thus, efforts are primarily directed at society as the focus of change. This model has been rebuked by many practitioners as a result of difficulty in accurately pinpointing problematic areas and designating appropriate and realistic intervention methodologies. Effective intervention within the environment often is frustrating because it appears all-encompassing and lacks highly differentiated techniques. As more knowledge in identifying and modifying environmental variables becomes available, this approach becomes more feasible and acceptable.

The ecological perspective provides a useful framework for service delivery because it integrates intervention strategies that are people- , environment- , and transaction-oriented. The selection of any given strategy is based upon the threefold goal of improving the adaptive capacities of individuals, improving the supportive qualities of the environment, and improving transactions between people and their environments.[28]

The ecological concept of adaptation assumes that individuals are active and goal-seeking beings. As the world proceeds to change rapidly, individual efforts are involved in the dynamic process of adjusting, of attaining a satisfactory balance with the environment. While new options for attaining goals are created, some alternatives are simultaneously being eradicated. In order to maximize control over our lives, the ability to achieve a mutual interdependence is required. Outcomes of effective human interactions with the environment include personal competence, increased coping ability, a sense of relatedness/connectedness, autonomy, and identity.

An Example in Practice

One of the first attempts at utilizing an ecological approach in human services was manifested in the *therapeutic community* or *milieu therapy* model. Most often found in psychiatric settings, it is an effort to monitor systematically and to utilize every aspect of the environment, including human interactions among the staff and the patients on an around-the-clock basis. Each individual in the setting is expected to assume responsibility for the effectiveness of the community and to actively encourage optimal involvement. It recognizes the impact of the environment on the individual, the individual's capacity to act, and, in turn, to influence the environment; it also recognizes the results of various types of interactions between the environment and the individual. Therapeutic recreators often work as an important part of an interdisciplinary team in this type of setting.

Underlying Principles

The ecological perspective provides a structure for analyzing concepts and transactions. It is a generic model (a way of thinking) and therefore does not provide content. A profession (such as therapeutic recreation) contributes content in the form of values, goals, objectives, and professional knowledge. An ecological model can be perceived as a value-based systems orientation. While it can be applied to any field of endeavor (for example, social work, nursing, psychology, environmental design), it does assume fundamental principles. These principles are interpreted for therapeutic recreation and related leisure-services professionals:

> The relationship between the therapeutic recreator staff and the participant/client is based upon mutual respect and reciprocity, authenticity, and openness.
>
> While the total person—including current abilities, limitations, interests and needs—is recognized, progressive forces—those that enable individuals to move toward a state of well-being—provide a focal point for therapeutic recreation service delivery.
>
> Problems, liabilities, and deficits are a result of a multitude of variables. Single-factor causations are not helpful in understanding human behavior, faulty interactions, or inadequate environments.
>
> Individuals are concerned with issues of personal control and self-determination. Environments that are "least restrictive" and that provide maximum support are most helpful in enabling humans to attain a healthy interdependence with their environments.[29]

Goals of the Ecological Approach

The following goals comprise global purposes for therapeutic recreation services.

1. Maximize individual capabilities for growth and creative adaptation.
2. Increase the supportive properties of the environment.
3. Minimize the effects of individual limitations.
4. Reduce or eliminate environmental blocks and obstacles to growth and development.[30]

In consort with the above purposes, more defined goals of therapeutic recreation services can be clustered into three major categories.

Goals Directed Toward Individuals

Increase individual mastery in a social world.
Increase self-esteem.
Strengthen adaptive patterns.
Develop coping strategies.
Increase skills in social interaction.
Increase confidence and ability to assume control.
Develop interdependent functioning skills.
Increase degree to which the individual attributes personal success to own actions.

These goals are addressed in more depth in Chapters 5, 11, and 12.

Goals Directed Toward the Environment

Increase environmental opportunities for personal action.
Mobilize and support mutual aid systems, including personal networks, access to information, availability, and effective use of resources.
Increase the range of leisure services and opportunities available.
Educate identified groups within the community.
Design physical environments to support individual independence and human interaction.
Reduce architectural barriers.

These goals are addressed in more depth in Chapter 13.

Goals Directed Toward Interactive Processes

Facilitate change of interaction patterns in maladaptive situations.
Influence rearrangements within a given setting related to temporal and spatial design.
Connect people to resources.

Maximize impact of interactions based upon values of equality, mutual respect, and normalization.

Assist in integrating persons with and without disabilities.

Assist individuals in creating their own environments.

Chapters 9, 10, 11, and 12 will address these goals in more depth. All of the goals outlined above provide a basis for understanding what therapeutic recreators do. Refer to Figure 1–6.

If you have grasped the intent of this chapter, you will understand the following:

That persons with disabilities, regardless of the type or extent of the disability, have the right to human dignity; have the potential to grow, develop, and learn; and have the right to maximum participation in the community;

that the environment plays a major role in the ability of any individual to assume control over his or her own life and to possess maximum independence;

that the relationship between an individual and his or her environment is in flux;

that therapeutic recreation personnel need to address both the individual and the individual's environment that impacts upon his or her experience;

that the focus of our efforts (intervention) may be the individual, the environment, selected interactive processes—any or all of these.

One last note: The issues and processes introduced here and discussed throughout this text are geared toward a broad understanding of therapeutic recreation. However, you will find that these issues and processes are applicable to the entire field of leisure services. That is, intervention is not just limited to persons with illnesses and disabilities. Individuals who have no

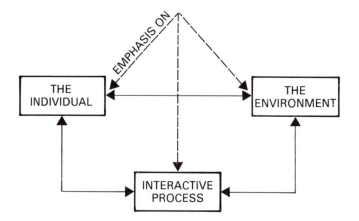

FIGURE 1–6 Concerns of Leisure/Therapeutic Recreation

identifiable or labeled medical condition are confronted daily with stressors that may affect their ability to have a harmonious relationship to themselves and their environments. Leisure service personnel are challenged to provide opportunities that maximize individual capabilities through supportive environments.

SUMMARY

This chapter introduced concepts that are the basis for the study of therapeutic recreation. Three major foundations of the field were identified, along with an overview of the evolution of thought within the therapeutic recreation profession.

We examined the interdependence of people and their environments from a social systems perspective. The major characteristics of social systems were presented, with their application to therapeutic recreation services. The concept of human ecology—a value-based perspective of systems—was explained, and the goals of therapeutic recreation using the ecological perspective were identified. This chapter also provided the organization for the remainder of the text.

DISCUSSION QUESTIONS

1-1. What factors have contributed to the increased awareness of persons with disabilities in our society? Which of these factors have had the most influence on your personally becoming aware of this sizable proportion of the population?

1-2. List at least four settings where therapeutic recreation (TR) services might be provided. Can you give a specific example of each of these in your own community?

1-3. Discuss briefly the importance of the three conceptual foundations to an understanding of therapeutic recreation:
       leisure, play, and recreation
       ideology toward persons with disabilities
       professional intervention

1-4. Define "social system" in your own words.

1-5. Identify two examples of systems from your own life and diagram them:
       a. Identify a system that has you as its main focus—in other words, what are the subcomponents that make you up?
       b. Identify a system that has you as a subcomponent.
       c. What happens when there is a change in a subcomponent of one of these systems? Can you think of an example of change occurring in these systems as a result of a change in a subcomponent?

1-6.   What is meant by "input, process, output, and feedback"? Give examples.

1-7.   What are some of the goals of therapeutic recreation? Use the ecological model to identify these goals.

NOTES

1. "Recreation: A $244 Billion Market," *U.S. News and World Report,* Vol. XCI, No. 6, August 10, 1981, p. 61.

2. Seppo E. Iso-Ahola, *The Social-Psychology of Leisure and Recreation* (Dubuque, Iowa: Wm. C. Brown, 1980); Gary Ellis and Peter A. Witt, *The Leisure Diagnostic Battery: Background, Conceptualization, and Structure* (Denton, Tex.: Division of Recreation and Leisure Studies, North Texas State University, 1981); John Neulinger, *The Psychology of Leisure* (Springfield, Ill.: Chas. C Thomas, 1974).

3. Ellis and Witt, *Leisure Diagnostic Battery,* p. 2.

4. J. Nina Lieberman, *Playfulness: Its Relationship to Imagination and Creativity* (New York: Academic Press, 1977).

5. Lynn A. Barnett, "Cognitive Correlates of Playful Behavior," *Leisure Today: Play, Journal of Physical Education and Recreation* (JOPER), October 1979, 40–43; Lieberman, *Playfulness;* Jean Piaget, *Play, Dreams and Imagination in Childhood* (New York: W. W. Norton & Co., Inc., 1962).

6. Iso-Ahola, *Social-Psychology of Leisure and Recreation.*

7. Michael J. Ellis, *Why People Play* (Englewood Cliffs, N.J.: Prentice-Hall, 1973); M. Czikszentmihalyi, *Beyond Boredom and Anxiety* (San Francisco: Jossey-Bass, 1975).

8. C. Forrest McDowell, *Leisure Wellness* (Eugene, Oreg.: Sun Moon Press, 1983).

9. "Remarks of the President to the White House Conference," *Programs for the Handicapped,* July 20, 1977, p. 3.

10. Wolf Wolfensberger, *The Principle of Normalization in Human Services* (Toronto: National Institute on Mental Retardation, 1972), p. 7.

11. Virginia Frye and Martha Peters, *Therapeutic Recreation: Its Theory, Philosophy, and Practice* (Harrisburg, Penn.: Stackpole Books, 1972), p. 41.

12. National Therapeutic Recreation Society (NTRS), "Philosophical Position Statement of the NTRS" (Alexandria, Va.: National Recreation and Park Association, 1982).

13. Ibid.

14. David R. Austin, *Therapeutic Recreation: Processes and Techniques* (New York, NY: John Wiley & Sons, 1982), pp. 59–60.

15. Marcia Carter, Glen E. Van Andel, and Gary M. Robb, *Therapeutic Recreation: A Practical Approach* (St. Louis, Missouri: Times Mirror/Mosby College Pub., 1985), p. 16.

16. American Therapeutic Recreation Association, *ATRA Newsletter* (Sand Springs, Okla.: ATRA, 1984).

17. William Ryan, *Blaming the Victim* (New York: Vintage Books, 1976).

18. Walter Buckley, *Sociology and Modern Systems Theory* (Englewood Cliffs, N.J.: Prentice-Hall, 1967), p. 41.

19. Ralph E. Anderson and Irl Carter, *Human Behavior in the Social Systems Approach,* 2nd ed. (New York: Aldine Publishing Co., 1978), p. 10.

20. Arthur Koestler, *The Act of Creation* (New York: Dell, 1967), p. 112.

21. Naomi Brill, *Working with People: The Helping Process* (Philadelphia: J. B. Lippincott, 1973), p. 64.

22. Ibid., p. 66.

23. Ibid., p. 66.

24. James F. Murphy, John Williams, E. William Niepoth, and Paul D. Brown, *Leisure-Service Delivery System: A Modern Perspective* (Philadelphia: Lea & Febiger, 1973), p. 1.

25. Ibid., pp. 1–5.

26. James F. Murphy and Dennis R. Howard, *Delivery of Community Leisure Services: An Holistic Approach* (Philadelphia: Lea & Febiger, 1977), p. 121.

27. Carel Germain, ed., *Social Work Practice: People and Environment, An Ecological Perspective* (N.Y.: Columbia University Press, 1979), p. 7.

28. Ibid., p. 17.

29. Ibid., pp. 7–20.

30. Ibid., p. 17.

THERAPEUTIC RECREATION CHANGE AGENTS

An image occurs to me: the ocean shore. An outcropping of rock extending into the sea, strong and narrow. Which, when I restrict my field of vision sufficiently, appears to split the water into two distinct and separate bodies. The action of the waves lapping up on either side makes it seem as though these two are ever straining toward one another, striving with each surge to overcome this rock which prevents their joining. . . . When, by simply stepping back and seeing more, by taking all-encompassing perspective, expanding consciousness, I see that the separation is only an illusion—that both waves are and always were part of the one ocean, separated only by choice of my perception and my motion of striving to be one. . . . [1]

INTRODUCTION

The image described above can be applied to the therapeutic recreation profession. As discussed in Chapter 1, the ecological perspective is useful in integrating two positions of intervention currently in practice: the clinical model and the social reform/community development model. The challenge facing therapeutic recreation specialists is to be able to step back and see both positions in a new way and, perhaps, as an integrated whole, by examining ourselves and our actions as therapeutic recreators. We are part of the system even though we may function in different settings and environments. Our inherent nature has an impact on the services we provide.

Service roles and functions imply action. As we integrate the practice of therapeutic recreation and recognize the evolutionary and adaptive nature of people and their environments, we can begin to intervene more effectively and improve the interaction that takes place between the two. We will begin to take action that results in an improved sense of relatedness and connectedness not only to the people we serve and their living environments, but also to each other as professional colleagues. The place to begin is to examine who we really are, the nature of our actions, and how this may affect our effectiveness as agents of change. This challenge stirs the heart and mind to new patterns of thought and behavior. It requires courage, confidence, and a willingness to explore.

The ecological perspective of service delivery is a multifaceted approach. In this model, service providers are seen as change agents. This implies that we not only act to stimulate the development of individuals but we intervene within the community as a whole. This intervention enables us to improve the transactions between the individual and the environment. If this concept of growth and change is to become a reality, it is imperative that we no longer just adapt to existing organizational and social systems and maintain traditional service roles. We are challenged to expand our roles to implement innovative functions that respond to the dynamic needs of individuals and their environments.

In order for us to understand our potential to become change agents, we need to ask ourselves the following questions:

1. Can a service provider act as a catalyst and effectively intervene and enable individuals to bring about desired changes that may promote their growth and development?
2. Can a service provider act as a community organizer and effectively intervene and enable communities to bring about desired changes?
3. Can the role of the service provider be expanded to include the process of facilitating the dynamics of planned social change?

THE NEED FOR CHANGE

As therapeutic recreation professionals expand their roles to include the facilitation of the dynamics of planned change, we stimulate society to take responsibility for the alienation of some of its citizens. In order to help an individual grow and develop, the community in which that individual lives must accept and respect individual differences. As service providers, we examine the barriers in the community that prevent people from being independent before assuming that individuals with disabilities may need specialized services.

Starting with Self

Challenging expectations are ascribed to us within this ecological intervention approach. We need to assess our values and human characteristics that will be relevant to our role as a change agent. Understanding the characteristics of effective change agents, which includes knowing our basic value structures, is an important consideration to the success of this approach. Generally speaking, we need to be creative, sensitive, honest, perceptive, and have the ability to communicate the need for change in our services and the community. These action-oriented skills involve an element of risk. Our life experiences provide a strong foundation upon which we can enhance ourselves and take the necessary risks to relate to the individuals we serve and their environments. We can assume the professional functions of change agents described throughout this book if we are aware of our potential to learn, to grow, and to change.

HUMAN EFFECTIVENESS

Several models of human effectiveness will be discussed briefly in this chapter. They are presented as a framework to assess our personal and professional effectiveness. One theme that recurs throughout this chapter is the notion that service providers need some basis upon which to conceptualize higher levels of human functioning. Assuming that if service providers have an increased awareness of attitudes, perceptions, motives, goals, needs, self-concept, and level of human functioning, they will have the potential to be effective change agents. Another assumption that needs to be stated is that the same concepts and constructs of intervention (individual and environmental) that apply to facilitating individual and community change can also apply to stimulating change in the service provider.

Behavioral theorists, such as Maslow, Allport, Rogers, and Blocher, have developed human effectiveness models. Maslow developed an holistic-dynamic theory of human motivation. In this theory, human development is conceptualized as a process through which human needs are satisfied and human potentialities realized. Maslow arranged human needs in a hierarchical structure in an ascending order. This hierarchy includes physiological needs, safety needs, belongingness and love needs, esteem needs, and self-actualization needs.[2] The higher-level needs will emerge only when lower-level needs have been satisfied.

Another model of human effectiveness that can be applied to a service provider is Gordon Allport's *mature personality*.[3] This author developed a composite model of psychological maturity characterized by six distinct criteria. These criteria describe an individual who consistently reaches out to people, is sensitive, consistent, and concerned about human beings and their participation in community living. The mature personality reflects an individual who is concerned about enhancing the quality of life.

Carl Rogers' model of human effectiveness, the *fully functioning person*, evolved from his own theoretical orientation and clinical experience.[4] He identified three characteristic qualities involved in the process of becoming a fully functioning person. The first quality involves an openness to experience. A person in touch with this quality is not defensive or resistant to the environment or to change. The person has accurate and realistic perceptions of self and the environment. The second characteristic quality of the process is *existential living*. Rogers defines this aspect of experiencing life as an ongoing process. During this phase of the process there is absence of rigidity and imposed structure. The third quality of the person involved in this process, according to Rogers, appears to be an increased ability to trust oneself. Rogers explains that human feelings are utilized as a trustworthy guide to behavior.

Donald Blocher, in an attempt to synthesize some of the ideas presented in the human effectiveness models conceptualized by Maslow, Allport, and Rogers, developed the concept of the *effective personality*.[5] Blocher describes five clusters of behavior identified as characteristics of the effective personality. According to Blocher, an individual with an effective personality is one who is consistent, committed, controlled, competent, and creative.

These models of human effectiveness form a basis for conceptualizing an optimum level of human development. A service provider who strives to reach and operate at the highest level of human development has the potential to become an effective change agent. The professional who strives to operate at this level of human effectiveness can begin to accelerate changes within a community, which may enhance the acceptance of human differences and the realization of human potential.

SUPPLEMENTAL ELEMENTS OF HUMAN EFFECTIVENESS

In addition to the human effectiveness models presented above, other behavioral theorists have identified singular elements of human effectiveness. Considering all the aspects of human effectiveness is important in order to understand fully the inherent qualities necessary for change agents.

Authenticity

An additional characteristic of an effective service provider or change agent is *authenticity*. Being authentic in relationships with the person being served, with colleagues, and with other service providers denotes honesty, sincerity, and openness. The change agent is a role model for the individual recipient of services, and if service providers are authentic in their relationships with participants, then the enabling action they facilitate will have a positive, growth-enhancing impact on the participant.

The idea of the "transparent self," articulated by Sidney Jourard, best describes the quality of authenticity. The author suggests that authenticity means

. . . dropping pretense, defenses and duplicity. It means an end to playing it cool, an end to using one's behavior as a gambit designed to disarm the other fellow, to get him to reveal himself before you disclose yourself to him.[6]

In other words, the quality of a transparent self, according to Jourard, is the ability to reveal one's self fully to another.

Self-Renewal

The concept of *self-renewal*, as a form of planned change in organization development, has been addressed by Paul Buchanan. Self-renewal refers to a condition attained by an organization through a process of development. An organization achieves self-renewal when it becomes

. . . sufficiently viable to continuously adapt to its changing environment and its own internal forces. . . . It becomes a system or framework within which continuous innovation, renewal, and rebirth can occur.[7]

One condition that may affect the reality of self-renewal within an organization is the effectiveness of the workers within the organization. Buchanan explains that when workers realize that their role relations are ineffective, they have the opportunity and responsibility to change their role relations in order to enhance effective performance. When this development occurs, according to Buchanan, the workers must have

. . . the freedom—as well as the obligation, the knowledge, the skill, and the organizational climate—required to devise more effective practices. And this freedom means, in part, room for diverse views—for pluralism.[8]

This concept of self-renewal can also be interpreted as a characteristic of human effectiveness. The professional's role as a change agent should be characterized by innovation, renewal, and rebirth. When these processes are inherent characteristics of the service providers, they may be able to adapt more readily to the growing needs of individuals and their environments as well as encourage innovation, renewal, and rebirth with the individual and the community.

One way to illustrate innovation, renewal, and rebirth is by means of a cycle. For example, consider two types of services planned and delivered to individuals with disabilities: segregated and integrated. Figure 2–1 illustrates these services and places them into an holistic context. As the needs of individual recipients of services change, recipients are able to move into a type of service to meet their specific needs and interests. As a community becomes more open and responsive, its members are able to accept and include a wide variety of people with various abilities. This fluid process is possible because the service providers are constantly designing new strategies, renewing their commitments, and experiencing change. The service provider is also

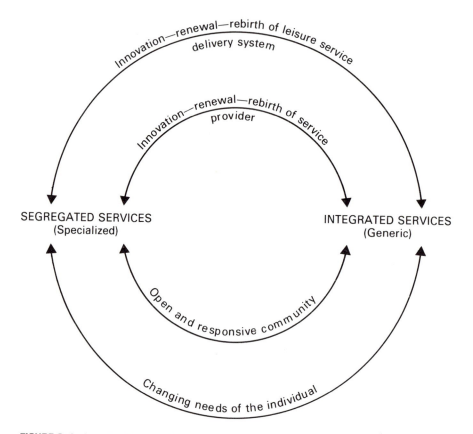

FIGURE 2-1 Innovation-Renewal-Rebirth: An Holistic Cycle

acting as a catalyst by enabling a leisure service delivery system to do the same. This holistic cycle can be applied to different variables that are affected by innovation, renewal, and rebirth.

The most important factor to remember about the concept of innovation-renewal-rebirth is that it is dealing with whole persons and systems. It places individuals and communities into a holistic context, a cyclical life process.

Role Adaptability

The change agent may need to employ diverse types of interventions to facilitate optimum development when working with individuals and communities. However, not all professionals will be able to assume all service roles with equal effectiveness. Service providers must be aware of the variety of service roles and perhaps look to others who are more effective in different roles. According to Blocher, Dustin, and Dugan

> The personal characteristic emphasized here, flexibility, is the ability to shift from one role to assume another. The change agent needs to assess the situation to make accurate diagnosis about the system as he fills the role of a social scientist. At the same time he will engage in many intense interpersonal relationships.[9]

Change agents involved in relationships with consumers and their communities require a degree of freedom within relationships to respond to their own perceptions and impulses. This freedom accords the change agent

> . . . the greatest opportunity to grow emotionally and personally and to contribute maximally to the same kind of growth in others. Unfortunately, in many social systems, the role opportunities are limiting and the role expectations so constricting that little opportunity for personal and emotional growth exists. . . . The construct of role adaptability as a property of a social system implies that some degree of role freedom exists and that role conceptions and role expectations are matters open to continuous inspections, discussion, and negotiation.[10]

Creativity

Creativity is dependent upon flexibility and adaptability. Compromises constantly come into play in any change effort, and finding an agreeable compromise between the ideal and the real is difficult. One key in overcoming this barrier is to remember that compromise and negotiation do not have to imply weakness or a win-lose situation. Progress can be made in change efforts when organizers put flexibility and adaptability into practice. Actively applying these skills unleashes our ability to solve problems in a creative manner.

Our multifaceted profession is often called upon to identify problems and determine possible solutions. The ability to do this depends upon our experience and technical skills. Each community is different and possesses its unique characteristics and problems. Likewise, solutions will also need to vary. What works in one community may not work in another.

How can we determine the best solution? Is there really only one solution to any problem? If we try something that doesn't work, does it mean that the problem cannot be solved? The *best* response to these and similar questions is *creativity*. Creative thinking is a process, and when it is applied it unlocks our ability to see entirely different perspectives. Creativity helps us to realize that there are many solutions to one problem. Each human being has the potential to look at a situation, analyze it, and think something different.

Why should we be creative? Ideas are born, nurtured, implemented, and eventually die. This is a reality and a characteristic of life. Life implies change and change produces growth. Roger von Oech, a creative-thinking consultant, suggests two reasons why we should be creative. He states:

> The first is change. When new information comes into existence and circumstances change, it's no longer possible to solve today's problems with yesterday's solutions. Over and over again, people are finding out that what worked two years ago won't work next week. This gives them a choice. They can either bemoan the fact that things aren't as easy as they used to be, or they can use their creative abilities to find new answers, new solutions and new ideas.
>
> A second reason for generating new ideas is that it's a lot of fun. As a matter of fact, I like to think of creative thinking as the "sex of our mental lives." Ideas, like organisms, have a life cycle. They are born, they develop and they die. Creative thinking is that means, and like its biological counterpart, it is pleasurable.[11]

The above message seems playful in nature and certainly blends with our understanding of the leisure experience. Change strategies designed with this in mind have the potential of having healing effects and speeding up the process of recovering from the effects of change. Laughter and play are powerful tools that recreators can naturally apply in difficult situations.

Another perspective on the importance of creativity comes from a person with a unique experience. The writer Norman Cousins stimulates a deep level of moral thinking, and he shares a valuable lesson he has learned from his experiences and explorations:

> The most important thing I have learned is that one of the prime elements of human uniqueness is the ability to create and exercise new options. The ultimate test of education is whether it makes people comfortable in the presence of options; which is to say, whether it enables them to pursue their possibilities with confidence. Similarly, a society can be judged according to the number and range of options of consequence it makes open to its people. What an individual decides to do with his or her life; the mobility of people, ideas and goods; what a person believes or doesn't believe about the great mysteries of life; how people are to be represented in their individual and collective needs and desires—all these involve the options that otherwise go by the name of natural rights.[12]

Creativity, like most concepts, possesses many different meanings and interpretations, and defining concepts is usually our first step in developing understanding. The following definitions of creativity and creative thinking are offered as a stimulus to explore this concept and reflect upon its meaning.

George Prince offers a series of definitions of creativity that suggests dichotomy.

> Creativity: an arbitrary harmony, an expected astonishment, a habitual revelation, a familiar surprise, a generous selfishness, an unexpected certainty, a formable stubbornness, a vital triviality, a disciplined freedom, an intoxicating

steadiness, a repeated initiation, a difficult delight, a predictable gamble, an ephemeral solidity, a unifying difference, a demanding satisfier, a miraculous expectation, an accustomed amazement.[13]

Gerard Nierenberg provides a general, working definition of creative thinking that includes its outcome.

Creative thinking, broadly defined, means coming up with something new. It is part of human skills thinking. These are the skills that have insured human survival, therefore cultural continuum (civilization) and growth.[14]

Barriers to Creative Thinking

As with most things in life, there exist barriers to creative thinking. We begin this discussion in a creative manner by looking at barriers or problems in a new way. Rather than perceiving barriers or problems in a negative manner, we can change our perspective and look at problems as unsolved opportunities. When we do this we are able to see something very different. We find ourselves changing our attitude. If we reflect for a moment on our personal experiences we can be sure that in most situations in which there has been conflict it is almost always an attitude that was the basis of our conflict or perception—and that we can change.

Creative thinking requires an attitude or outlook which allows you to search for ideas and manipulate your knowledge and experience. With this outlook you try various approaches, first one, then another, often not getting anywhere. You use crazy, foolish, and impractical ideas as stepping stones to practical new ideas. You break the rules occasionally, and hunt for ideas in unusual outside places. In short, by adopting a creative outlook you open yourself up to both new possibilities and to change.[15]

One central theme occurs throughout the literature of creativity—that is, that the search and development of our creativity is found internally. We all have the capacity to think in creative ways if we allow ourselves to be open to this experience. George Prince explains that creativity requires practice and patience with ourselves. The author remarks:

The practice of creativity must begin with yourself. You obtain the greatest leverage by investing time and thought in making more and better use of the talent you now own. The first step is to become even more sensitive to the problems that surround you. Each problem is an opportunity to exercise, develop and test your skill. Tackle each one you see—privately at first. In each case you first collect extensive data within yourself. These include facts, opinions, feelings, and even seemingly irrelevant material. Second, you use this data as a launching pad for loose speculating. You use your wit and energy to search out and pursue the possibly useful rather than pick out and concentrate on flaws. Only in season do you give formal recognition to shortcomings, and even then they are identified as something to be overcome.[16]

CARE FOR THE CARE GIVER

As therapeutic recreators we are members of the helping professions. As a result we are prime candidates for the negative effects of job-related stress. We may experience physical, mental, and emotional strain on a daily basis. The human-service professions are associated with certain characteristics that increase our vulnerability to the negative effects of stress (headaches, backaches, indigestion, hypertension, fatigue, insomnia, and so forth). Greenberg and Valletutti have clearly identified some of the characteristics of human-service professionals. These characteristics are applicable to therapeutic recreators. The authors suggest that, in general, human-service professionals

1. Become deeply involved in the lives and well-being of others, whether they are clients, patients, students, or congregants.
2. Wield some degree of control in directing the activities of others.
3. Are regularly exposed to human grief, deprivation, struggle, and failure, as well as the inability of others to cope adequately with their daily functions—mental, physical, or emotional.
4. Spend long, usually irregular, hours accomplishing specific job tasks.
5. Are expected to or expect to perform a variety of activities, many of which may not be directly related to his or her specific function.
6. Are expected to be familiar with and able to make referrals to a variety of resource agencies.[17]

It is not our purpose here to explore in depth the nature of stress or outline specific strategies to deal with its impact. The authors' intent is simply to point out the susceptibility to the effects of stress that we all experience. Many resources are available on stress management. However, the authors reinforce the belief of experts in stress management that human-service professionals who understand the causes of stress, its relationship to physical and mental illness, and the techniques for reducing it may be able to avoid job burnout. Stress reduction techniques such as creative visualization, exercise, nutrition, biofeedback, and meditation are a few coping strategies that may prevent the negative effects of stress. These techniques are worthy of exploration by any professional who wishes to design a program suited to his or her needs.

TRADITIONAL ROLES OF THE SERVICE PROVIDER

As the concepts and principles of therapeutic recreation have developed, the role of the specialist has changed and broadened. Some of these roles include administrator, supervisor, leader, educator, therapist, counselor, consultant, community educator, advocate, leisure educator, facilitator, and researcher. It is evident that the functions of therapeutic recreators are diverse and vary depending on the type of service, setting, and the purpose and goals of the organization and institution in which the services are rendered.

The continuum model developed by Gunn and Peterson identified service roles in terms of the nature of the interaction between the individual and the service provider.[18] Compton and Witt identified service roles in terms of their effectiveness in the delivery of leisure services.[19]

RECONCEPTUALIZED FUNCTIONS OF THE SERVICE PROVIDER

The traditional roles of service providers have changed over the past decade. Therapeutic recreators have traditionally been functioning as ancillaries who operate from the periphery of the system. Our service roles and functions are still developing in terms of their effectiveness in making the process of integration a reality because we have been unable to intervene consistently to change the very systems that produce the problems or barriers that we are expected to alleviate. Reconceptualizing the function of the service provider from the traditional perspective to change agents will serve to extend service providers into their social systems.

Role functions, broader and more flexible in scope, enable individuals with disabilities to realize their full potential, keep their dreams alive, and promote accessible, patient, supportive, and challenging communities. The uncertain adventure of community living can be an environment for change when it is open and responsive.

Therapeutic recreation specialists who first and foremost perceive their role only as "therapists" may have difficulty being effective change agents.

> When any field of endeavour becomes highly professionalized, a host of unforeseen problems are created. Consider the "process" of enhancing one's status with highly valued medical model symbols—for example, "therapeutic recreation" and "recreation for special populations." In an attempt to gain dignity and acceptance, professionals have accepted, perhaps unconsciously, the medical model and segregationist attitudes which have restricted recreation and leisure experiences for devalued persons for so long.[20]

John Gliedman dynamically stresses the effect a therapeutic orientation has had on an oppressed minority in our society. The author suggests:

> For society at large, the "therapeutic state" (to recall Nicholas N. Kittrie's term) is a threat, not a reality. But millions of disabled Americans already live within the invisible walls of a therapeutic society. In this society of the "sick," there is no place for the ordinary hallmarks of a present or future adult identity, no place for choice between competing moralities, no place for politics, no place for work, and no place for sexuality. All political, legal, and ethical issues are transformed into questions of disease and health, deviance and normal adjust-

ment, proper and improper "management" of the disability. To recall political scientist Sheldon S. Wolin's fine phrase, the "sublimation of politics" has proceeded furthest of all with handicapped people. Of all America's oppressed groups, only the handicapped have been so fully disenfranchised in the name of health.[21]

The attitudes change agents bring into relationships with the people they serve and with the community may affect their role opportunities and expectations. Change agents, in whatever role they find themselves, must relate to service recipients with a conviction that they are first and foremost individuals with dignity and worth, with the freedom of choosing their own alternatives for growth.

A change agent can be perceived as a person who encourages other people and the community they live in to make favorable changes. Change agents acknowledge that the people they are involved with are ultimately responsible for changing themselves. From this perspective, change agents recognize that change is a developmental process and that they are participants in the process.[22]

TABLE 2-1   Attitudes of the Change Agent Implementing the Process of Intervention and Facilitating Individual and Community Change

BELIEFS AND ATTITUDES ABOUT INDIVIDUALS WITH DISABILITIES	BELIEFS AND ATTITUDES ABOUT RECREATION SERVICES AND RECREATION PROFESSIONALS	BELIEFS AND ATTITUDES ABOUT THE PROCESS OF INTERVENTION
Respects and values the worth and dignity of every human being.	Recognizes that a therapeutic recreation specialist who is first and foremost a "therapist" is not suited to be an effective community change agent.	Believes that intervention is a developmental process that involves individual skill development and the elimination of barriers that hinder independence.
Believes that individuals with disabilities, regardless of the severity, have inherent abilities and human rights.	Believes that a full continuum of services should be available and accessible to all people in the community.	Believes that service delivery systems should be coordinated to make the most effective use of existing and emerging community resources.
Believes that individuals with disabilities should participate in every level of leisure service delivery systems and other community structures.	Believes that leisure service delivery systems should move toward such value-based principles as normalization, individualized lifestyle, and self-determined decision making.	Believes that the problems to be faced in intervention are system problems; that structures, policies, procedures, and attitudes must be changed to enhance the quality of communities and individual lifestyles.

Generic and therapeutic recreation professionals who are reluctant to reshape their approach may be resistant to changing their service delivery systems. Therefore, change agents need more than just a mastery of facts regarding disabling conditions, programming, community organization, and social change. Service providers functioning as change agents need to acquire basic attitudes toward others, the profession, and the process of intervention in order to be most effective in the process of planned change.

Donald Fessler has identified basic attitudes appropriate to the effective change agent.[23] He describes an individual who accepts the complexity of life situations; acknowledges the related experiences of others; develops a broad understanding of their chosen profession; shows empathy and compassion for others; affirms an ultimate objective to facilitate change; helps people accept unpleasant situations that cannot be changed; accepts personal limitations; does not use a leadership role for personal gain; helps others to make personal sacrifices for the common good; and values other people's time as much as personal time.[24]

Table 2–1 identifies beliefs and attitudes that are necessary for a change agent to implement the process of intervention.

REGISTRATION/CERTIFICATION OF THERAPEUTIC RECREATORS

The professionalization of therapeutic recreation has been a developmental process. The attributes of this process include professional training, credentialing (registration, certification/licensure), standards of practice, and a philosophical position statement. The registration/certification programs available to therapeutic recreation personnel are voluntary in nature.

These registration/certification plans have undergone adjustments in their criteria, all of which are designed to upgrade and recognize appropriate professional training and education of those providing therapeutic recreation services. Through the efforts of state and national professional organizations, there exist registration/certification programs. The issue of licensure, however, is still being examined. As one author observes: The "present registration criteria for therapeutic recreators have become more critical to hiring and retention of personnel and to the development of a nationally recognized credentialing program for therapeutic recreation personnel."[25]

SUMMARY

The characteristics of service providers are just as important as the skills they demonstrate when providing services. This chapter encouraged us to examine our qualities as people in relation to becoming a therapeutic recreator.

Service providers who believe in an ideology of human dignity and demonstrate a self-caring attitude toward themselves will be effective in their roles as a change agent.

Throughout this chapter we learned of the need to broaden our professional functions to increase our effectiveness in service delivery and community change. The service provider is essential to intervention strategies with both individuals and communities. Our ability to grow as individuals is directly related to our ability to encourage and facilitate that growth and zest for life in others and their communities.

DISCUSSION QUESTIONS

2-1. Why is an understanding of oneself important in working with other people, particularly with clients/consumers?

2-2. What are some personal characteristics that are important to possess and refine as professionals?

2-3. What does it mean to be a *change agent*?

2-4. How will you prevent "burnout" in your own professional life?

2-5. Interview two therapeutic recreation specialists from the same community: one from a clinical setting, the other from a community setting. Talk to them about their job roles and how they function within the organization in which they are employed. How do their roles differ? How are they the same? How do they cooperate with other therapeutic recreation specialists in their organization, community, or within professional organizations? Have they been effective in bringing about change in relation to the individuals they serve, their organization, their community?

NOTES

1. Marilyn Ferguson, *The Aquarian Conspiracy: Personal and Social Transformation in the 80's* (Boston: Houghton Mifflin Co., 1980), p. 381.

2. A. H. Maslow, *Motivation and Personality* (New York: Harper & Row, 1970), pp. 35–47.

3. Gordon W. Allport, *Personality and Social Encounter* (Boston: Beacon Press, 1960), p. 162.

4. Carl R. Rogers, *On Becoming a Person* (Boston: Houghton Mifflin Co., 1961), pp. 187–189.

5. Donald Blocher, *Developmental Counseling*, 2nd ed. (New York: Ronald Press, 1974), pp. 97–98.

6. Sidney M. Jourard, *The Transparent Self* (New York: Van Nostrand Reinhold, 1971), p. 133.

7. Paul C. Buchanan, "The Concept of Organizational Development, or Self-Renewal, as a Form of Planned Change," in *Concepts for Social Change*, ed. Goodwin Watson (Washington, D.C.: COPED, National Training Laboratories, N.E.A., 1967), p. 2.

8. Ibid., p. 3.

9. Donald Blocher, E. Richard Dustin, and Willis E. Dugan, *Guidance Systems* (New York: Ronald Press, 1971), p. 301.

10. Ibid., p. 133.

11. Roger von Oech, *A Whack on the Side of the Head* (Menlo Park, Calif.: Creative Think, 1982), p. 5.

12. Norman Cousins, *Human Options* (New York: Berkley Publishing Corp., 1981), p. 17.

13. George M. Prince, *The Practice of Creativity* (New York: Macmillan Publishing Co., 1970), p. xiii.

14. Gerard I. Nierenberg, *The Art of Creative Thinking* (New York: Simon & Schuster, 1982), p. 12.

15. von Oech, *Side of the Head*, p. 6.

16. Prince, *Creativity*, p. 201.

17. Sheldon Greenberg and Peter J. Valletutti, *Stress and the Helping Professions* (Baltimore, Md.: Paul H. Brookes Publishers, 1980), pp. 5-6.

18. Scout Gunn and Carol Peterson, *Therapeutic Recreation Program Design: Principles and Procedures* (Englewood Cliffs, N.J.: Prentice-Hall, 1984), pp. 10-26.

19. David Compton and Peter Witt, "A Philosophical Statement of the National Therapeutic Recreation Society, A Branch of the National Park and Recreation Association," (Arlington, Va., NRPA, Mimeo paper, 1979).

20. Peggy Hutchison and John Lord, *Recreation Integration* (Ottawa, Ontario: Leisurability Publications, 1979), p. 20.

21. John Gliedman, "The Wheelchair Rebellion," *Psychology Today*, August 1979, p. 101.

22. William W. Biddle, *The Community Development Process* (New York: Holt, Rinehart & Winston, 1965), p. 270.

23. Donald R. Fessler, *Facilitating Community Change: A Basic Guide* (La Jolla, Calif.: University Associates, 1976).

24. Ibid., pp. 32-35.

25. Marcia Jean Carter, "Registration of Therapeutic Recreators: Standards from 1956 to Present," *Therapeutic Recreation Journal*, Vol. XV, No. 2 (Second Quarter 1981), 17-18.

MEANINGS
OF LEISURE
AND WELL-BEING

You knock, then enter the room of Martha L., a woman who has recently been admitted into a short-term (90 day) rehabilitation program for drug-dependent adults. You are well prepared for this initial conversation, as you have read all of the available information on the new resident. You introduce yourself and indicate that you are on the staff of the recreation therapy department.

"What next?" is the reply. "I sure don't need any more therapy. . . . And what's this about my leisure? I have more free time than I need or want! Don't bother me, thank you!"

Well, you *thought* you were ready. What you think of as positive and rewarding is apparently seen from another perspective by Martha. Is it a matter of terminology? What do the terms *recreation* and *leisure* mean to her?

INTRODUCTION

Leisure: A Complex Phenomenon

It is simultaneously
    a personal expression,
        a way of perceiving life,
        an avenue to self-knowledge,
        an opportunity for personal growth and development;
    a social force,
        part of the fabric of community life,
        a link to society, our heritage and culture;

> an economic determinant,
>   an expensive undertaking,
>   a free afternoon;
>   a reflection of who we, as a people, are.

Define what leisure means to you personally. For each of us, the definition will be just a little different. The differences result from our individual histories, beliefs, exposure to options, social groupings and interactions, and a multitude of other psychological, social, and environmental factors. Through the work of leisure scholars, we have seen several major leisure "concepts" emerge, which account for most of these perspectives of leisure.

Because leisure services that are based on different perspectives are delivered differently, it is important to first have an understanding of these various perspectives. Further, these major concepts need to be examined in the context of disability.

Remember—the term *leisure* (play, recreation) means different things to different people. The following section reviews leisure concepts and some of their implications for service delivery.

CONCEPTS OF LEISURE

Leisure as Time

"It's my free time, generally on weekends, after I'm done studying, working at the restaurant, and when the apartment has been cleaned." This personal interpretation reflects the concept of leisure as time or "free time." (Remember Martha.) It was described by Charles Brightbill, a prominent educator and writer, as ". . . time beyond that which is required for existence, the things which we must do to make a living . . . discretionary time, the time to be used according to our own judgment or choice."[1]

In addition to time left over, a second component of this definition stresses individual choice. This quantitative concept of leisure has been popular because of its seeming neatness. Many leisure service delivery systems have been based upon it, providing the bulk of programs during well-defined periods of the day (after work) and the week (weekends) for consumption "at the discretion" of the beholder. Intertwined with this concept is that one may deserve leisure after work. In fact, the concept of discretionary time evolved out of the industrialization of society.

The implications for a "free time" approach to leisure services for ill or disabled persons are multiple. This group as a whole faces severe underemployment and unemployment conditions, resulting in financial constraints that tend to limit participation in desired experiences. Leisure, defined as time left over from work, then may have little meaning. In fact, seen from this perspective, disabled persons may not "qualify" for leisure and its potential benefits. The "freedom" underlying free time and freely chosen ways to enjoy that time may be minimal.

On the other hand, disabled individuals often have an abundance of nonobligated time. In the past, recreation activities have been used almost exclusively to fill this time, whether or not the experience was chosen or desired by the consumer. For many adults in particular, this has resulted in a dehumanizing, derogatory experience. Free time or "forced leisure" that was imposed more by a society that offered few meaningful options of any kind to disabled persons became a negative force with detrimental consequences. Of course, one would have to ask if this is really leisure at all.

A critic of the discretionary time perspective, James F. Murphy, suggested that the "bankrupt, philosophical and operational perspective of the recreation and park movement—discretionary time" does not reflect the reality or the potential of consumers.[2] It only serves to further fragment and compartmentalize the lives of individuals who are looking for ways of integrating their lives and connecting with their environment. This approach to service delivery probably quite unconsciously minimizes interaction between disabled and able-bodied individuals. Recreation programs in public settings serving the disabled during the weekday minimizes opportunities for integration and provides a subtle message that recreation is diversionary, even custodial, meant to keep people busy and to prevent them from further deterioration.

The *custodial* service delivery model, an outgrowth of the discretionary model, still exists in some settings. Its emphasis is on providing activities with the intent of diverting the consumer and reducing boredom. It is, of course, an outdated and often dehumanizing approach to service delivery.

Leisure as a Behavioral Function

The concept of leisure as a behavioral function suggests that preference for participation in certain kinds of leisure experiences is contingent upon one's characteristics and life conditions. Those socioeconomic characteristics, such as race, occupation, and social class, once thought to be significant in predicting leisure behavior, while still important, appear to be less reliable indicators in an age of advanced technology.[3] If we consider the increasing pluralistic nature of society (the diversity in lifestyles, the aging of the population, a diffusion of values via the media, increased mobility, the infusion of new cultural trends, and changes in demographic patterns), it is not surprising that these characteristics are not the only factors to consider in understanding leisure patterns. One of the best demographic predictors of leisure behavior is education.[4]

Little research has been undertaken in regard to disability and its relationship to leisure behavior. Compton and colleagues conducted a study of the recreation behavior and attitudes of 1,679 veterans in Veteran's Administration Hospitals across the country. They reported that as the length of hospitalization increased, individuals tended to show more negative signs of institutionalization. Persons hospitalized for longer periods reported a higher degree of external locus of control and extrinsic motivation than those hospitalized for a shorter period of time. They also found that individuals who are older and more disabled, and those hospitalized longer, perceived more barriers to leisure than their younger, less-disabled and short-term hospital peers.[5]

The existence of a disability has often been associated with selected activities. What kinds of activities are associated with people who are mentally retarded, visually impaired, or who have cerebral palsy? Answers such as the Special Olympics, arts and crafts (particularly caning and basket weaving), and bowling have all been promoted for these respective "groups." However, the result is the creation of a stereotype; that is, one that links specific activities with specific disabilities, often to the exclusion of other experiences. Therapeutic recreation and related leisure service personnel must examine carefully the premises underlying practices that *limit* people's experiences and their development.

Exposure to any experience is a prerequisite for voluntary selection of that experience. The more individuals are made aware of the myriad leisure options and are provided the freedom to try new things, even if they are risky, the more likely a true leisure experience will result. Further, associating certain activities with certain individuals, based upon the existence of a disability, would seem to hinder the potential for interaction outside of the specific disability group.

One outgrowth of this perspective is the *activity* model used mostly in institutional settings, such as nursing homes, some hospitals, and state schools. This approach to services leans heavily on the provision of a range of activities for the residents. Program calendars are filled with everything from volleyball to movies to arts and crafts. While some personnel make these activities as meaningful as possible, in many places the activities serve merely to fill time. They keep people from becoming overly bored and from getting "in the way."

Therapeutic recreation has reached a level of sophistication where we now know that the activity per se is relatively unimportant. It is what happens to an individual during the process of engaging in the activity that is important.

Leisure as a State of Mind

The concept of leisure as a state of mind—as discussed by Kelley, Murphy, Neulinger, and other prominent researchers—stresses the perceptions, the attitudes, the feelings, and the needs of the individual. It is not the time period or the specific behavior or activity that defines leisure, but the individual who defines what it means to be at leisure. DeGrazia explained this perspective as "a state of being, a condition of man."[6]

Need-satisfaction has been studied as the basis for leisure, and this has promoted the theory that the behavior of individuals is based upon a hierarchy of needs. Individuals engage in selected experiences to meet specific needs. Identifying *why* people participate in a given activity, attend a specific event, or interact with particular social groups may help us to understand leisure better. The "meaning" of the experience, as identified by the perceiver (participant), is central to this formulation.

The concept also implies that the "person at leisure" has personal freedom: freedom of choice, freedom to move about at will; and a general lack of constraints, be they physical, psychological, or environmental. These conditions, apparently central to leisure, are often denied or missing in the lives of disabled individuals, who have often been constrained because of personal limitations and, more often, social policies. Progress in the area of new technical devices, such as communication and mobility appliances, compact kidney dialysis, and insulin pocket machines, as well as advances in social awareness, providing equal access to all settings and range of behaviors, should contribute to even more freedom.

Social-Psychological Perspectives

> Social influence, which is the key concept in social-psychological analysis, is said to occur whenever one individual responds to the actual, imagined or implied presence of one or more others.[7]

Thus states Seppo Iso-Ahola, a leading researcher in leisure studies. Within the theoretical framework of this perspective, an individual and a social component are at work. The emphasis is on understanding recreation and leisure behavior in the context of dynamic interactions between a given individual and other individuals, groups, or cultural elements. This contemporary thinking proposes that behavior is the result of a changing person in a changing world.[8]

While the many variables affecting leisure from this perspective cannot be covered here (see Iso-Ahola, 1980), several major determinants of leisure behavior will be reviewed.

Iso-Ahola suggests that leisure service practitioners should be concerned with enhancing individual participants' "perceived freedom, perceived competence, social interaction, and other intrinsic rewards."[9]

> Perceived freedom is high when a person attributes the initiation of leisure behavior to self, but it is low when he ascribes the source of behavior to external factors.[10]

People tend to select leisure experiences in which they can expect a reasonable level of success, for expectations are often based upon past experience and past success. This perceived competence is reflected in statements such as "I like to play tennis because I am good at it." This tennis player is apt to perceive that his or her good shots are a result of personal ability, and that poor shots are a result of external factors, such as a pitted court surface, sun in the eyes, or a competitor who is even more competent.

Perceived freedom and perceived competence form a core for another determinant of leisure behavior, namely *intrinsic motivation.* When an activity is engaged in for its own value, the behavior is said to be intrinsically motivated. When a person participates in that same experience for an external reward, it is considered to be extrinsically motivated. Intrinsic motivation is enhanced when a person attributes leisure participation to perceived competence.[11] While this factor plays a major role in defining leisure to the individual, Iso-Ahola reminds us that intrinsic motivation operates in a social milieu and not a vacuum. There is evidence that those experiences in which we freely choose and in which we see ourselves as competent are governed by external factors, such as cultural values, norms, and sanctions.[12]

Many people also define perceived competence in terms of skills in interpersonal relationships. If one considers the phenomenal support of spectator sports, or the importance of a substantial audience at a concert or play, then the importance of others' participation in some leisure activities is obvious. In fact, one of the most important reasons for leisure participation is social interaction.[13]

The *cause* of an individual's leisure behavior is also of concern to therapeutic recreation personnel. The *attribution theory* embodies the principles related to the causal analysis of behavior.

> Attribution refers to the process by which a person (either an actor or an observer) obtains information about an act and then makes causal inferences about the source of that act.[14]

Sources are considered to be internal (related to the individual's personality) or external (situational, environmental). People have a tendency to analyze the causes of their own behavior and the behavior of others perhaps in an attempt to make sense out of the world. Perceiving causes of behavior, whether correct or not, is one way that individuals exercise control over their environment.[15]

What is the importance of this perspective to therapeutic recreation service providers? The *ecological service delivery model* is closely aligned to the social-psychological perspective of leisure. As introduced in Chapter 1, this model assumes that there is a dynamic exchange of energy (information, values) between individuals and their environment. An understanding of this concept of leisure, then, is fundamental when applying this service delivery model to both therapeutic recreation and broader leisure services. For example, let us first consider the concept of perceived freedom. While that is a relative factor (who, after all, is totally free to do exactly as he or she wishes?), some individuals, such as those with disabilities, may experience additional constraints, be they the result of physical limitations, architectural barriers, or the attitudes of others. In some instances, such as in hospitals, institutions, and other long-term care facilities, the personal freedom of patients is extremely limited, if not nonexistent. This is manifested by room and bed assignments, rigidly scheduled routines on a 24-hour basis, predetermined daily activities, and controlled personal interactions. While this represents an extreme, it does in fact exist to some degree in many settings. Iso-Ahola reports on several studies examining the effect of personal control and freedom on elderly, institutionalized persons. The data he reviewed indicated that an increase in the perceived personal control of residents enhanced their activeness, interpersonal activity, mental alertness, and psychological well-being. In contrast, individuals in nursing homes who were not given opportunities for personal choice were found to have a higher mortality rate.[16] Apparently the less perceived control the individual experienced, the more the feeling of helplessness resulted. Perceived personal control can be enhanced by providing the individual with opportunities to make meaningful decisions in everyday living.

Increased perceived competence, resulting from the attainment of new leisure skills, seems to enhance self-concept. Exposing consumers to new leisure experiences and encouraging them to develop more advanced skills in familiar activities is helpful in building self-concept. Because consumers can attribute competence either to themselves or to the environment, they should be given sufficient feedback to increase their attribution to themselves.

Labeling people also has an effect on causal attribution. Severance and Gasstrom studied the causal attributions for persons labeled mentally retarded. Observers perceived that the performance failure of subjects was due to their lack of ability, while attributing successful performance of these individuals to effort.[17] This perception, repeated frequently, could result in *learned helplessness,* that is, the inability of the individual to believe that he or she can control events and behaviors. This perception is reflected in the statement, "It doesn't matter what I do, it won't work."

Sometimes personality traits are viewed as causing behavior. Disability, for example, may be perceived as a primary characteristic that has related role requirements and behaviors. The "mentally retarded personality" or the "personality of blind persons" was not an uncommon phrase some time back. This stereotype bolsters the perception that it is the disability that causes the deviance and failure, and that external factors bring success. This, again, promotes learned helplessness.

Iso-Ahola suggests that the main task of therapeutic recreation is "to increase patients' perceived control and mastery over the environment (assist them in making internal attributions) and to prevent them from inferring helplessness."[18]

Therapeutic recreators can encourage individuals to develop new skills and heighten their sense of competence. If consumers learn socially acceptable leisure behaviors and activities (nonstereotypic), they are likely to increase the attribution to themselves, and observers are likely to attribute success to that person's competence. Thus, leisure skills and behaviors can be a powerful tool for minimizing disability stereotypes and for enhancing the public's perceptions of persons with disabilities.

Intrinsic motivation is one of the key dimensions underlying the delivery of therapeutic recreation. Several models that stress the development of intrinsic motivation by a person otherwise operating from an extrinsic modality will be discussed a little later in the chapter.

Lifestyle, Disability, and Leisure Behavior

Lifestyle is a term used to refer to an individual's pattern of behavior. According to Feldman and Thielbar, it is defined as:

1. a group phenomenon, influenced by a person's participation in various social groups;
2. it pervades many aspects of life and spills over into many areas of social contact, e.g., work, play, school, family, church, etc.;
3. it implies a central life interest in which a single activity (avocational pursuits, work, religion, cultural heritage, etc.) pervades a person's other interests and unrelated activities.[19]

This concept has significance because it represents a complex perspective upon which to analyze leisure behavior. As a social phenomenon, one's lifestyle affects or is affected by social groups, including family.

While it would be ridiculous to suggest that there is a "disability lifestyle," the existence of disability is apt to have an effect upon lifestyle. For those individuals who are independent, disability may have a very limited impact. That is, the lifestyle of a musician or a ski buff may be possible and desirable. For others, the range of what might be considered possible lifestyles may be curtailed as a result of financial, social, medical, and other restrictions. Central life activities may not be personally chosen, and social groups may be imposed. As more options become available to disabled individuals, lifestyle will take on new meanings.

The awareness of available leisure resources and options can make an important contribution to the development of a satisfactory lifestyle. The *education/counseling model* focuses on the development of individual skills, particularly as they relate to leisure behavior. Educational and counseling strategies are employed to encourage self-awareness and independence. This orientation may be incorporated into a range of settings, from a rehabilitation hospital to a school to the community. Recreational activities are among the educational methods used to facilitate the development of skills. Services provided under this model may be called *leisure education* or *therapeutic recreation*. The processes used will be examined in Chapter 12.

Leisure as a Social Instrument

The use of a picnic to bring factory workers together to form a union . . . a "Summer-Fun-for-All Festival" to encourage persons with and without disabilities to share in creative play experiences together . . . a neighborhood carnival that addresses street crime. . . . These are all examples of the use of a leisure experience or recreation activity as a means (instrument) to achieve another end. James Murphy described the social instrument orientation as a "threshold" to desired ends, be it racial equality, improved motor performance, or social integration.[20] Recreation is, in fact, often used as a way to reach other objectives. High-risk outdoor games, such as those used with Ropes Course and Outward Bound Programs, have been used with predelinquent youth and business executives alike to help build group trust and cohesion and to increase self-confidence. The use of recreation activities to facilitate change regardless of the target of the change strategy provides the essence of this concept. Understandably, this orientation to leisure is useful in analyzing approaches to therapeutic recreation services.

The *clinical/rehabilitation/therapy model* follows the medical intervention model. Recreation activities are used as a tool to improve functional behavior, to develop personal skills, and/or to facilitate coping and adjustment behaviors. This orientation is found primarily in clinical settings in which medical personnel assume a primary helping role, although offshoots of this concept are found in some nonmedical settings. This orientation to service delivery is often termed *recreation therapy*. The use of this rehabilitation model will be discussed more fully in Chapter 11.

Environmental Perspectives of Leisure

Many environmental factors, including actual settings, have been identified as being critical to understanding leisure behavior.

> Environmental settings or physical places tend to be identified by particular qualitative characteristics which relate to particular symbolic, ritualistic and/or functional meanings by various social groups.[21]

A taxonomy of leisure locales was developed by Cheek and Burch:

1. The specialized moral order, or the social value placed on a locale;
2. The physical design, which refers to the set-up and arrangement of a locale; and

3. The social structure, referring to the composition and social organization of the locale.[22]

Certainly, locales used by ill and/or more dependent disabled persons have multiple effects. A hospital environment, for example, may advance or hinder the efforts of the patient to progress or to cope. The use of hospital gowns with slit backs, side rails on beds, stainless steel and white surroundings emphasize the isolation of the patient from regular life patterns and interactions with family and friends. Conversely, a hospital environment can be made more tolerable by the availability of informal recreation areas, a sun porch, warm colors, and friendly, caring personnel. A building reserved exclusively for adults, labeled the Center for the Mentally Retarded, located on a street where several such "exclusive" facilities exist, carries certain social connotations. An aesthetically pleasing community center that is clean, well lighted, colorful, surrounded by landscaping and architecturally barrier free will likely elicit different reactions, carry different social messages, and entertain varied leisure responses from a community center that is littered, dark, and set among unkempt grounds.

The relationship between environment and behavior has blossomed into a whole field of study. Called *environmental psychology*, it analyzes the relationship between these two factors. Research indicates that environmental factors, such as aesthetics, influence psychological attitude. However, research regarding the interaction of environment and behavior in the context of disability is in its infancy. Although therapeutic recreation specialists are not expected to be experts in environmental psychology, they can be cognizant of the potential impact of specific factors on leisure behavior and maximize or minimize the impact of these factors, as appropriate and feasible. The concept of *normalization*, discussed in Chapter 9, provides a foundation for examining the impact of various types of environments, and their related messages, on persons with illnesses and disabilities.

Nurturance is another important facet of the environment. Nurturance includes both physical and human (social, emotional) support. A physically supportive design encourages positive interactions and is pleasing to the senses. An emotionally supportive environment encourages openness, trust, risk taking, social interactions, and caring. Again, the ecological model provides insight into the value of a supportive environment.

A Holistic Perspective of Leisure

A *holistic* perspective of leisure is one that recognizes and integrates multiple factors affecting leisure behavior. Social, psychological, economic, cultural, and personal and environmental variables are all thought to contribute to the leisure choices made by individuals and to the meanings that individuals attribute to leisure.[23]

This orientation would seem to hold much promise for the delivery of therapeutic recreation and related leisure services to ill and disabled persons and for understanding their leisure patterns. No longer would the existence of disability itself be the criterion upon which to base services. Rather, the total individual, along with his or her cultural, racial, and ethnic heritage; current life activities, personal goals, interests, needs, and abilities could be recognized within the matrix of environmental variables. Services that enabled the individual to derive inner satisfaction through maximum self-determination would be the primary goal. A range of service delivery options would recognize that individuals need different levels of support, be they physical, emotional, or social, during various phases of life in order to maximize self-determination.

A holistic perspective also serves to integrate different life spheres and to recognize that elements of leisure exist in all aspects of one's day-to-day life, not just in those hours away from work. Leisure, then, could potentially occur any time, any place, doing almost anything. This perspective is also reflected in the *ecological model* of service delivery.

The foregoing section suggests that therapeutic recreation and related leisure services that are based upon different leisure concepts "look" different. That is, they have different functions and, often, different strategies. While no one concept of leisure is "right," some perspectives, such as the sociopsychological and holistic models, provide a more defensible basis for the delivery of services. These reflect a view of life that is based upon integrating individual growth and development within complex and dynamic environmental forces.

Perhaps most important is the recognition that leisure provides the foundation for the delivery of therapeutic recreation services. Without an acknowledgment of the importance of leisure, there is no reason for delivering therapeutic recreation services, and without this acknowledgment, services would lack meaning.

THE FUNCTION OF PLAY AND RECREATION

"Living in a state of play means living more humanely," observes Joseph Levy in his opening statement of *Play Behavior.*[24] He continues:

> To be free, and therefore to know play (know thyself) means to realize simultaneously the supreme importance and utter insignificance of our existence. To play means to accept the paradox of pursuing what is at once essential and inconsequential. . . .
> Play, then, is necessary to affirm our lives. It is through experiencing play that we answer the puzzle of our existence.[25]

Psychologists, anthropologists, sociologists, leisure scholars, educators, and countless others have contributed to the growing literature on the phenomenon of play. Yet no universal answer has emerged to such questions as: "What is play?" "What causes play?" "What are the consequences of play?" Levy, however, identified three common characteristics of play in his extensive review of the literature: *intrinsic motivation, suspension of reality,* and *internal locus of control.*[26]

Intrinsic motivation. Levy suggests major implications of intrinsic motivation as related to recreation and mental health.

1. Intrinsic factors produce self-realization, self-actualization and self-esteem.
2. Satisfaction of the self-esteem needs leads to feelings of self-confidence, worth, strength, capability and adequacy.
3. Extrinsic factors are associated with . . . dissatisfaction and which constitute a negative, avoidance dimension.
4. Extrinsic factors are considered to prevent dissatisfaction but to have little effect in creating positive attitudes.
5. Similarly, the reduction of intrinsic factors may result in diminished satisfaction but not in the creation of dissatisfaction.
6. Recreation's key role in promoting mental health, therefore, is seen as lying in its potential for promoting and planning experiences which will contribute to the satisfaction of intrinsic needs. Similarly, mental illness and failure to find satisfying recreational activities that meet the intrinsic needs of the organism may be seen as closely related.
7. What is being postulated is that mental health and mental illness are two independent dimensions of adjustment with the degree of illness or health reflecting the individual's disposition toward primary satisfaction of extrinsic or intrinsic needs.[27]

What qualities characterize this concept of intrinsic motivation? Czikszentmihalyi[28] reported that individuals who are intricately, inextricably involved in a play activity experience a cohesion or convergence of their self-awareness with their behavior and the immediate environment. The momentary loss of self-awareness has been documented in several studies.[29] This phenomenon has been called the "flow" experience.

Personal involvement in a play experience and, thus, intrinsic motivation also tend to be enhanced by the processing of the maximum amount of relevant information and the blocking of stimuli irrelevant to the activity. The "optimal flow of information" is reflected in the ability of an athlete to shut out external information—such as the cheering crowd, cameras, and the harassment of opponents—when attempting to make a critical point at the end of a game.

Suspension of reality. Transcending reality allows us to retreat from physical, social, and emotional pressures. Through play, escape to fantasy is accepted. In this state, we can test ourselves utlimately. We create our own world.

Internal locus of control.   This concept was also discussed under "perceived freedom" in leisure. Constructed from Rotter's social learning theory,[30] people who are internally motivated believe that they have responsibility and control over their own lives. This element is a central feature of most literature that attempts to explain play.

In an effort to illustrate the relationship of intrinsic/extrinsic motivation, suspension of reality, and the internal locus of control in play, Levy developed the model shown in Figure 3–1. As one engages in purer forms of play behavior, intrinsic motivation, the suspension of reality and internal locus of control increases. Simultaneously, the player's individuality unfolds. The person becomes more of who he or she is.

Antecedents to Play

In order for play to occur, certain conditions (antecedents) must exist. For example, the player must possess the requisite cognitive, social, motor, and affective skills needed to participate in any given experience. Further, the ability to play is linked directly to the individual's physiological and emotional functioning. The use of unnatural substances such as drugs, alcohol, cigarettes, tranquilizers, and sedatives that alter the body's physiology will alter the play experience.

Again, we recognize the impact of the environment on the player. Stories abound about the supposedly exotic play behavior (for example, hot tubs, windsurfing, sunbathing on the beaches, hot-air ballooning, hang gliding, and so forth) of Californians. The weather is an obvious factor in these activities;

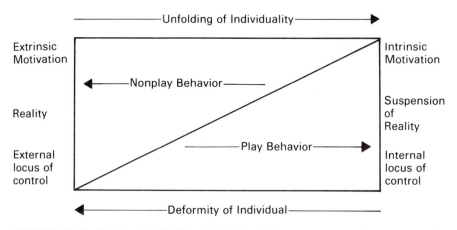

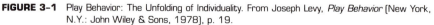

FIGURE 3–1   Play Behavior: The Unfolding of Individuality. From Joseph Levy, *Play Behavior* [New York, N.Y.: John Wiley & Sons, 1978], p. 19.

it not only allows such behavior to occur but it encourages outdoor activity much of the year.

Other environmental variables, such as amount of air and water pollution, noise level, textures, colors, scents, and spatial dimensions (crowdedness, open space), have all been identified as factors in leisure patterns.

Consequences of Play

Researchers from many disciplines have reported the results of play activity, particularly with children. Dr. Lynn Barnett, a prominent leisure scholar, has reported the cognitive benefits of play for small children. She suggests that play provides the medium by which children understand their world and become familiar with their environments. Further, she suggests that play contributes to problem-solving ability and divergent thought processes.[31]

Other research has shown play to be a precursor to creativity and abstract thinking. Other well-known benefits include social and language development, mastery over the environment, and individual growth. The immense potency of play within our lives is just beginning to be understood. Therapeutic recreation and other leisure service personnel have a serious responsibility to understand the complexity of this phenomenon and to strive to enhance it in every way possible in the lives of those people we serve.

Levy has proposed a paradigm that suggests the relationships between important components of play. This is illustrated in Figure 3-2. The reader should note that the person, the environment, and the interaction among them serves as a foundation for his model.

The Play-Therapy Continuum

When play is discussed in the literature in context of disability, the concept of *play as therapy* predominates. This concept has become so popular that "play therapy" has evolved as a separate entity within the field of counseling. It presupposes that because play (toys, role playing/drama) is a natural form of self-expression for children, it can be used to diagnose and treat children, particularly those with emotional disorders. Children drawn into playful experiences are observed for their behaviors under various conditions. For example, given a task that they find frustrating, how do children react? Shown puppets that might be symbolic of a family member, what kind of emotion is exhibited? Of course, the more externally controlled, the more extrinsic, and more reality-based the experience, the less playful the experience will be, according to Levy's model.

The purpose of therapeutic recreation is intricately intertwined with the play-therapy dichotomy. For individuals whose mental, physical, and social functioning is severely impaired, recreation is often used as a tool for assisting them in developing maximum functioning capabilities. (Recall the

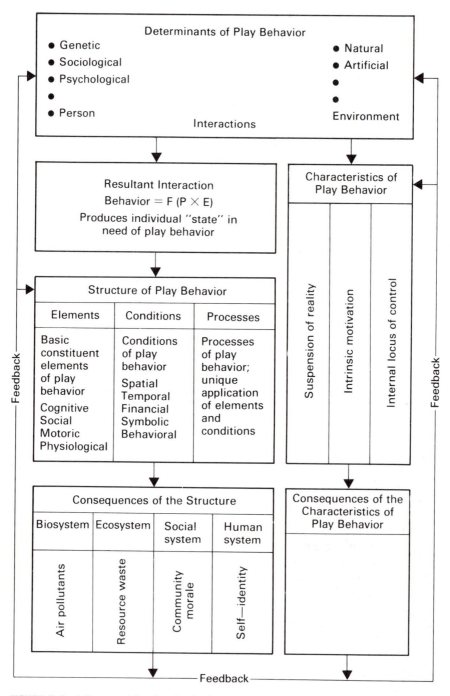

FIGURE 3-2 A Conceptual Paradigm for the Study of Play Behavior. From Joseph Levy, *Play Behavior* [New York, N.Y.: John Wiley & Sons, 1978], p. 58.

rehabilitation model.) For Peter, a severely retarded youngster with minimal social interaction skills, this might mean that a therapeutic recreator would initially call Peter's name, using physical cues to attain eye contact before rolling a ball to him. Eventually, two or three other youngsters might join in the ballgame. In this instance, the game, the setting, the players, and the strategies for "playing" the game are all selected by the therapeutic recreator with a specific purpose in mind. The players may be reminded to "look," to "roll the ball," and to attend (focus on) to a variety of social skills. Rewards for "appropriate" or desired behavior may include food, such as fruit; a smile; clapping and other individually tailored acknowledgments. It is evident that the experience is focused on skill development in the here-and-now; the service provider is in full control, and the rewards are external, received after selected displays of behavior. Although a game provides the medium, the experience is therapeutic if it indeed responds to the needs of the individuals involved. The behaviors are not necessarily reflective of play.

Let us use the above example. While the "game" is in progress, two other youngsters indicate that they want to join in. After a few minutes, they are laughing joyously at their successful and not-so-successful attempts at catching, rolling, throwing the ball within the group. They concentrate on the ball and try some new ways of tossing the object. For them the experience is different. They chose to play and have a degree of control in the game. They are also encouraged to focus more on the game itself than on any specific behaviors, and their primary reward stems from being involved in the game although the attention given by the therapeutic recreator remains important. This experience could be perceived as more playful.

Several leaders in the field of therapeutic recreation have contributed to its conceptual development by offering continua that show individual movement from a therapy to play experience.

Edith Ball outlined a series of four sequential steps through which a person could progress to reach a truly "recreative state." These steps are shown in Table 3–1.[32]

TABLE 3–1 Recreative Progression

EXPERIENCE	TYPE OF TIME	MAJOR MOTIVATION
1 Activity for sake of activity	Obligated time	Drive is outer directed
2 Recreation education	Obligated time	Drive is outer directed
3 Therapeutic recreation	Unobligated time	Motivation is inner directed but choice of experiences is limited
4 Recreation	Unobligated time	Motivation is inner directed

Source: Edith L. Ball, "The Meaning of Therapeutic Recreation," *Therapeutic Recreation Journal*, 4:1, 1970, p. 18.

Note that the nature of the experience, the source of motivation, and the time are basic elements identified by Ball. The first step could be considered a diversionary/custodial phase.

A much later therapeutic recreation continuum was presented by Peterson and Gunn in their important contribution to the field. From a synthesis of the literature existing through the mid-1970s, they clustered therapeutic recreation services into three major areas: rehabilitation, leisure education/counseling, and recreation participation. This model, reproduced in Figure 3-3, served as a basis for the philosophical statement accepted by the National Therapeutic Recreation Society (see Chapter 8).

Note the concepts of obligation and freedom included in the Peterson and Gunn model. Does this resemble Levy's model? Also note that the *function* of service delivery changes as the individual changes. That is, as the individual gains freedom from internal constraints and external obligation, the role of the therapeutic recreator changes from therapist to educator to leader. It is important to remember that not all individuals who are ill or disabled go through all phases of the model. Many, in fact, will not be in need or will not desire therapeutic recreation services. For those whose conditions indicate such a need, they may participate in two or all three phases simultaneously, or never use some of the phases.

Locus of Control

The Gunn and Peterson model also delineates another important aspect of service delivery—the consumer-professional relationship. The notion of *locus of control* refers to the balance of authority and responsibility within a specified relationship. In a helper-client relationship, the ultimate goal is to transfer authority for decision making from the helper to the client.

Other leaders in the field have attempted to explain the nature of this relationship. Berryman, quoted in Frye and Peters' classic on therapeutic recreation, contributed a model that depicts recreation activities as "experiential bonds" between the service provider and the consumer. Berryman used the analogy of the DNA molecule to explain how the service provider uses the activity to connect a person more to his or her environment, thus assuming more control of one's personal behavior.[33]

In an adaptation of a model proposed by Tannebaum and Schmidt, Frye and Peters discussed the authority–freedom dimension inherent in therapeutic relationships.[34] Figure 3-4 illustrates these steps.

1. The recreator administers a highly structured program under medical orders.
2. The recreator "sells" the program to the patient and motivates the patient to participate.
3. The recreator and patient construct a program together.
4. The recreator advises the patient and the community.
5. The patient is free to participate in any activity available to him or her.

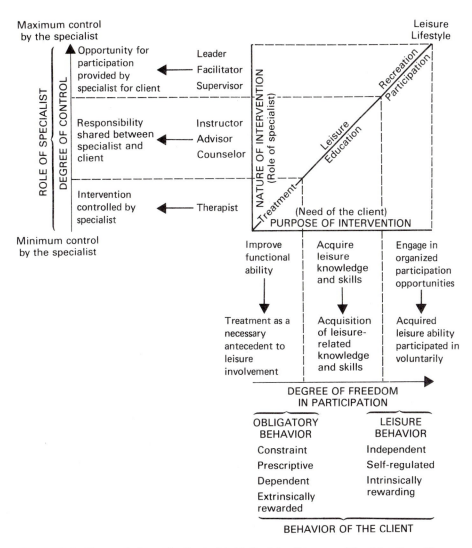

FIGURE 3–3 Therapeutic Recreation Service Model. Carol Ann Peterson and Scout Lee Gunn, *Therapeutic Recreation Program Design: Principles and Procedures,* 2nd ed. [Englewood Cliffs, N.J.: Prentice-Hall, 1984], p. 44.

Each of these models emphasizes the dynamic consumer-professional relationship inherent in the process of the individual developing, gaining skills, and acquiring confidence.

Perhaps one of the harshest criticisms leveled at health and human-service professionals by consumer advocates centers around this issue of au-

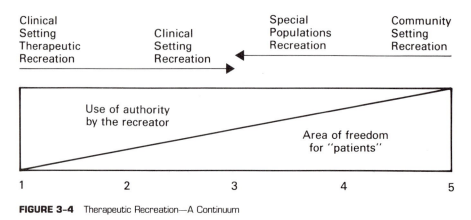

FIGURE 3-4   Therapeutic Recreation—A Continuum

thority, responsibility, and control. While no one would claim that individuals consciously enter helping professions so that they can control others, it is suggested that the process of becoming "professional" may be antithetical to the actual liberating process. Does sitting in the class you are now attending and reading this book contribute to students turning into professionals who have a difficult time relinquishing control over those they are apparently attempting to assist? We each must confront this question honestly and repeatedly. Does the process of becoming prepared to be a helper, of taking tests to be recognized and certified in a helping field, somehow influence our ability to allow consumers to take charge of their own life? Under what conditions are we most effective or least effective in empowering people, in enhancing their capacity for self-determination, and in maximizing their ability to make decisions from among meaningful alternatives? This, perhaps is one of the most serious questions we must deal with as professionals and one that provides a fulcrum for professional ethics.

One of our great challenges is to learn how this process of individual change (assuming responsibility for self, assuming control over one's environment) takes place and to develop more effective strategies for encouraging independence, decision making, and other important leisure and life skills. One of the goals of therapeutic recreation is to provide skills that enable people to play and to be as self-determined as possible. A consumer's ability to play, then, should never be contingent on the presence of a service provider. Perhaps one of the best indicators of independence is an individual's creativity, playfulness, and spontaneity without immediate encouragement or guidance from a leisure professional. A major aim of any services we provide is to have the foresight to assist individuals in achieving skills that will be of benefit beyond the parameters of the service itself.

HEALTH AND WELLNESS

Basic to the practice of allied health professionals, including therapeutic recreation specialists, is the goal of health. Health is a relative concept, defined by culture, society, and the individual. For example, Jack, who experiences continual back pain, proceeds through daily activities including work and play. Jack's family and friends are barely aware of his pain. He has learned to cope with and even control the pain. Joe also experiences continual back pain. He often interrupts his daily activities and focuses on the pain in an attempt to relieve it. Joe's family and friends are constantly aware of his discomfort. These individuals have experienced, perceived, and defined a similar condition quite differently. They may be said to have different toleration levels of pain.

Society plays a crucial role in how individuals perceive health and illness. One only has to visit the local pharmacy or the "health" section of the supermarket to see the hundreds of products aimed at relieving pain. Manufacturers of these products spend immense sums in marketing their wares to consumers.

From a broader perspective, we have been cautioned about the hazards of food additives and certain food products. Greasy, fried foods and white sugar top the list of foods certain to trigger unpleasant effects. Certainly we know about the potentially lethal effects of cigarette smoking; the dangers of chemicals in our foods; drugs, including alcohol; and pollutants in the air and water.

The popularity of physical activity continues to grow, with bicycling, swimming, jogging, and innumerable forms of activity consuming more of our effort. Business again has capitalized on this health movement by trying to outfit us in designer sportswear, shoes, wristwatches, and radios. Ample evidence exists that large segments of our society are very health conscious.

Culture is also a determinant in health promotion. Whereas middle- and upper-class white Americans tend to dominate participation in the activities mentioned above, blacks, Hispanics, Asians, and other racial and ethnic groups participate less frequently. Thus, as leisure service providers, if we are to promote health-oriented leisure experiences, we must understand the preferences and practices of people from diverse backgrounds.

Wellness and Illness

The concept of *wellness* has broadened the scope of our definition of "health" in the last few years. It is a dynamic dimension that affects every aspect of life, and it is affected by both internal and external variables. Wellness is much broader than the "absence of disease." In a holistic sense, it refers to one's entire organism: the integration of one's physical, mental, emotional, spiritual, and social status. It is affected by nutrition, events in one's life, the nature of one's work, play, and living environment, including aesthetics, cleanliness, and interpersonal relationships. This holistic perspective toward health and therapeutic recreation practices will be examined more closely in Chapter 11.

Prevention and Cure

The concepts of health, wellness, prevention, and cure are critical to therapeutic recreation personnel. As professionals, we each interface constantly with consumers (and colleagues) who are dealing with various levels of stress, both eustress (positive) and distress (negative). Every person living in the hubbub of today's society is consciously or unconsciously trying to balance external and internal forces to maintain a state of homeostatis (balance). Therapeutic recreators often work in environments where people either are dealing with medical difficulties, are sick, or are considered sick either by themselves or someone else. (Remember that disability is often erroneously interpreted as illness. See Chapter 5).

Therapeutic recreation specialists have a unique role when it comes to promoting wellness. Rather than focusing on the illness or the disability per se, we emphasize *intact strengths.*

Leisure has long been recognized for its value in inhibiting human dysfunction. The wellness movement has provided support for the idea that satisfying leisure experiences contribute to physical, emotional, and mental well-being. Through recreation activity, healthful life rhythms, and interactions, disease-producing variables, such as the negative consequences of distress, can be counteracted.

The issue of personal control again arises in relationship to health. An active consumer awareness movement is reflected as consumers become proactive and assume a participatory role in taking care of themselves. Engaging in physical activity or choosing other leisure pursuits that are health-oriented (physically, mentally, socially, emotionally) is one way of empowering oneself, of using one's freedom. The connection between health and leisure, then, becomes more obvious.

Professional and popular literature both emphasize the role that one's mental state or attitude plays in contributing to health. If you reflect back on the section on leisure as a state of mind and some of the consequences of play activity, you will see another connection between leisure and wellness.

The Role of Humor in Well-Being

We are all familiar with the expression "Laughter is the best medicine." And we all know that momentary and wonderful sensation when something hits us as funny. Anything from a smile to a giggle to a rip-roaring, soul-filled laugh produces a sense of release. Norman Cousins shares with us the intense personal power he discovered in laughter that helped cure a fatal illness he incurred.[35]

Humor and laughter are becoming increasingly recognized for their role in healthy living. Our individuality, our uniqueness, our perspective on life, and our humanness are all expressed in our humor.

Allied health personnel have found humor serves several purposes in health care delivery. As a prognostic tool, it has been found valuable in predicting recovery from some illnesses.[36] Further, it is instrumental in promoting communication, establishing social relationships, and relieving anxiety.[37] In health care settings, where the tone is often serious and emotionally laden with fear, embarrassment, anxiety, sadness, or concern, humor hastens familiarity and serves as a vehicle for expressing selected messages. When usual social norms are violated, such as the invasion of privacy or the creation of dependence, laughter can help to break the tension. It can have a liberating effect on service providers and consumers alike by defusing negative emotions.[38]

In a three-year study at the University of Southern California, researchers found that laughter was effective in reversing the mental process of aging. Individuals in long-term facilities were better able to cope with their environments if daily activities could be enriched with humor.[39] Again, humor was found to result in a change of attitude.

In another study, humor was found to ease tension and smooth the social interactions of physically disabled and able-bodied individuals.[40]

Humor can take on many forms, from comedy, to clowning, to spontaneous play behavior, to creative art to —. Humor, as are leisure and health, is defined by society, by culture, and by the individual. What an American black finds funny, an American Indian might not. British and Australian humor often seems unhumorous to Americans. As we further understand the role of humor in promoting wellness, we must take into account differences in how people perceive it.

In sum, humor appears to be another link between leisure and wellness. That is, as humor promotes physical, social, mental, and emotional well-being, it enables an individual to experience a unity of being, an integration of parts, and a sense of connectedness with the environment. It is a powerful tool that, used with sensitivity, may provide the key that further unlocks the mysteries of humanity.

SUMMARY

Leisure was explored as a complex phenomenon, with varied determinants and manifestations. This chapter reviewed the major concepts of leisure and extended their implications for the delivery of leisure services within the context of disability.

The phenomenon of play and its major characteristics were discussed as they relate to the provision of therapeutic recreation. Health and wellness were explained as contributors to the delivery of leisure services.

This chapter provided an important foundation to help the reader better understand different professional and personal orientations to this field. How we deliver services—and the form that these services take—is directly related to given perspectives toward leisure, play, and health. The more we understand how they can be made operational, the more probable it is that our services do what we claim they do—that is, contribute to the quality of life within a community and enhance individuals' leisure functioning.

Finally, developing a strong conceptual basis for our service delivery is critical in the planning and designing of viable services. Understanding these concepts will also assist us in articulating the importance of our services to the public and to funders.

DISCUSSION QUESTIONS

3-1. There are many perspectives of the meaning of leisure. Each professional definition of leisure forms the basis for a type of service delivery model.

This chapter provides a brief overview of several major professional perspectives, their related service delivery models, and the potential/real implications for persons with disabilities. Identify some of the major characteristics of each perspective, and characteristics of the allied models, as they relate to disabled individuals.

Perspective	Model
Leisure as time	Discretionary/custodial
Leisure as behavior	Activity
Leisure from sociopsychological perspective	Ecological
Leisure lifestyle	Leisure education
Leisure as social instrument	Rehabilitation/therapy
Holistic	Ecological

3-2. Identify and briefly describe the three characteristics of play discussed by Levy.

3-3. Note that "locus of control" came up several times in this chapter. Define it and discuss its importance within therapeutic recreation service delivery.

3-4. Discuss the relationship between wellness and leisure.

Perhaps you can begin to see here that while the concepts discussed throughout this text have been traditionally related to people with disabilities, they also apply to those without disabilities.

CASE STUDY

Part I

The following paragraphs contain descriptions of existing therapeutic recreation programs. In small groups, read each one and respond to the following:

1. What leisure concept(s) does it embrace?
2. What service delivery model(s) does it embrace?
3. Would you want to be a participant in the program if you were a patient/client in this setting?

Activities are the prime concern of the Recreation Department. Therapeutic activities, whether group or individually oriented, are an integral part of the patient's rehabilitation to social and community life. With the assistance of volunteers, recreation therapy provides a meaningful use of leisure time with programs that include music sing-alongs, arts and crafts, field outings, bingo, sports, and table games.

The primary goal of the Recreation Therapy Division is to utilize recreational and functional techniques as part of the rehabilitation process. These techniques include helping a disabled person learn to live and enjoy a life in a society filled with physical and functional barriers. The staff plans each program to encourage the patient to reach his or her highest level of functional capability. Ultimately, independence in leisure activities is the major goal. The patient's previous recreational interests are rekindled whenever possible, or new activities are introduced.

Part II

Using your small group as a therapeutic recreation staff within either a rehabilitation setting or within a community parks and recreation setting, develop a description of a therapeutic recreation program. Use the concepts of leisure and their related service delivery models as a basis for a sound description. Perhaps you want to think about a setting where you have worked or with which you are familiar to help you develop this description. Consider how you would want a program to look if you were a patient or client in that facility; use this as a guide in developing this description. Share your group's descriptions in class.

NOTES

1. Charles Brightbill, *The Challenge of Leisure* (Englewood Cliffs, N.J.: Prentice-Hall, 1960), p. 4.

2. James F. Murphy, "An Enabling Approach to Leisure Service Delivery," in *Recreation and Leisure: Issues in Era of Change,*

eds. Thomas L. Goodale and Peter A. Witt (State College, Penn.: Venture Publishing, 1980), p. 197.

3. James F. Murphy, *Concepts of Leisure*, 2nd ed. (Englewood Cliffs, N.J.: Prentice-Hall, 1981), p. 135.

4. Ibid., p. 139.

5. Leisure Systems, "Survey of Recreation Attitudes, Preferences, and Interests of Veterans: Final Report," (Denton, Tex. and Columbia, Miss.: January 1982), pp. 40–41.

6. Sebastian de Grazia, *Of Time, Work and Leisure* (Garden City, N.Y.: Doubleday, 1964), p. 5.

7. Seppo E. Iso-Ahola, *The Social Psychology of Leisure and Recreation* (Dubuque, Ia.: Wm. C. Brown, 1980), p. 15.

8. Ibid., p. 186.

9. Ibid., p. 244.

10. Ibid., p. 186.

11. Ibid., p. 232.

12. Ibid., p. 236.

13. Ibid., p. 242.

14. Ibid., p. 215.

15. Ibid., pp. 215–216.

16. Ibid., p. 344.

17. L. J. Severance and L. L. Gasstrom, "Effects of the Label 'Mentally Retarded' in Causal Explanations for Success and Failure Outcomes," *American Journal of Mental Deficiency*, 81 (1977), 547–555.

18. Iso-Ahola, *Social Psychology*, p. 323.

19. Saul D. Feldman and Gerald W. Thielbar, eds., *Lifestyles: Diversity in American Society* (Boston: Little, Brown, 1972), pp. 1–3.

20. James F. Murphy, *Recreation and Leisure Services: A Humanistic Perspective* (Dubuque, Ia.: Wm. C. Brown, 1975), pp. 49, 129.

21. Murphy, *Concepts of Leisure*, p. 167.

22. Neil H. Cheek and Wm. R. Burch, *The Social Organization of Leisure in Human Society* (New York: Harper & Row, 1976), p. 155.

23. Murphy, *Concepts of Leisure*, pp. 179–191; Max Kaplan, as cited in Murphy, *Concepts of Leisure*, p. 179.

24. Joseph Levy, *Play Behavior* (New York: John Wiley & Sons, 1978), p. 1.

25. Ibid., p. 1.

26. Ibid., pp. 6–19.

27. Ibid., pp. 6–7.

28. Mihaly Czikszentmihalyi, *Flow: Studies of Enjoyment* (Chicago, Ill.: The University of Chicago Press, 1974).

29. Levy, *Play Behavior*, pp. 9–10.

30. J. B. Rotter, *Social Learning and Clinical Psychology* (Englewood Cliffs, N.J.: Prentice-Hall, 1954).

31. Lynn Barnett, "Cognitive Correlates of Playful Behavior," *Leisure Today* (AALR: JOPER, October 1979), 10–13.

32. Edith L. Ball, "The Meaning of Therapeutic Recreation," *Therapeutic Recreation Journal*, 4:1 (1970), 18.

33. Virginia Frye and Martha Peters, *Therapeutic Recreation: Its Theory, Philosophy, and Practice* (Harrisburg, Penn.: Stackpole Books, 1972), p. 43.

34. Ibid., p. 43.

35. Norman Cousins, *Anatomy of an Illness* (New York: W. W. Norton & Co., Inc., 1979).

36. Barbara Amy Cringle, "Humor Used As a Coping Mechanism by Adult Aphasics" (unpublished Master's thesis, San Jose State University, 1981), p. 1.

37. Vera Robinson, *Humor and the Health Professions* (Thorofare, N. J.: Charles B. Slack, 1977), p. 40.

38. W. F. Fry, *"The Impact of Mirth and Humor"* (abstract), American Psychological Association, Chicago, 1975.

39. Maxine Ewers, *"Life Enrichment Through Humor in Long Term Care Facilities,"* USC: Andrus Gerontology Center, 1980.

40. H. Wilke, *"From the Viewpoint of the Disabled,"* Twelfth World Congress for Rehabilitation of Disabled, 1972, pp. 14–18.

4

PERSONS WITH DISABILITIES
A Balanced Perspective

I do not choose to be a common man. It is my right to be uncommon—if I can. I seek opportunity—not security. I do not wish to be a kept citizen, humbled and lulled by having the state look after me. I want to take the calculated risk; to dream and to build, to fail and to succeed. I refuse to barter incentive for a dole. I prefer the challenge of life to the guaranteed existence; the thrill of fulfillment to the state calm of Utopia. I will not trade freedom for beneficence nor my dignity for a handout. I will never cower before any master nor bend to any threat. It is my heritage to stand erect and unafraid; to think and act for myself, to enjoy the benefit of my creations and to face the world boldly and say, this I have done.[1]

INTRODUCTION

Over a period of several decades perceptions of individuals with disabilities have changed and evolved. This evolution of conceptual thought and approach to service delivery forms the foundation for responding to the needs of individuals with disabilities. This conceptual framework would not be complete without creating a balanced perspective of individuals with disabilities. This chapter will briefly discuss the traditional approach to human development and will outline a perspective of disability as a variation in the human condition—an approach integral to the conceptual foundation of this book.

Viewing and Focusing: A Whole Image

The viewfinder is perhaps one of the most important features of a camera. This part of a camera allows the photographer to ascertain whether or not an image is "in focus." Skilled photographers will make the necessary adjustments to their cameras in order to ensure that the object of their attention becomes one complete image.

The human brain, like the viewfinder on a camera, has the quality of being able to examine, evaluate, and draw conclusions. In essence, we have the ability to make adjustments in our way of thinking in order to look at an object, person, or experience in complete focus. When this happens, clear and steady images can be perceived.

This analogy presents a thought-provoking perspective on the way in which individuals with disabilities are often perceived. Perhaps a viewfinder is out of focus when it only sees the disability. When an object is out of focus, not only is the image divided horizontally but it is also distorted as a whole. A disability is only one characteristic of the overall makeup of an individual. When a disability becomes the center of attention and the other qualities of a human being are not in view, then it becomes impossible to perceive one complete and focused image.

All human beings have capabilities and aspirations. These inherent characteristics that distinguish human beings from the lower animals are valued in our society. This belief in the importance of every human being is based upon a foundation of optimism.

Centering on the "whole" human being—that is, the cognitive, affective, physical, social, and spiritual domains of a developing person—directs our attention to their capabilities, interests, individuality, and life experiences. However, these five domains of human behavior are often viewed in isolation. This traditional, segmented approach to the study of human development and behavior often fails to recognize the unique quality and potential of every human being.

> In many instances it is essential, especially for research purposes, to consider only one small segment of development in order to identify cause-effect relationships. However, the danger of this segmentation is that the focus of a discipline can become so narrow that the individual is seen as an interesting entity rather than a unique person. When a person exhibits a variation (alternative predictable behavior) or deviation (unpredictable or pathological behavior) from the norm, the practitioner (professionally trained person) from the appropriate discipline frequently concentrates so heavily on that one aspect of the client (person needing assistance) that the other more normal aspects may be ignored. In other words, the practitioner may fail to recognize the client's strengths while trying to remedy his weaknesses.[2]

This segmented approach to the study of human development and behavior has not only had a limiting effect on various disciplines and their practitioners, but, more importantly, it has had a limiting effect on the lives of individuals with disabilities. Their so-called deviations have been diagnosed and studied. As a result, individuals with disabilities have been labeled; accordingly, segregated services have been planned for them.

This traditional approach to human development and behavior perceives disabling conditions as abnormal deviations. This view is often accepted and perpetuated without questioning and evaluating its historical impact on the lives of disabled people and the attitudes held by nondisabled people. One need not look very far to realize that many disabled people have been segregated on the basis of their disability label and perceived abnormality.

Focusing on a disabling condition may on one hand help us identify weaknesses and plan "appropriate" programs; on the other hand, this emphasis perpetuates an attitude of dependence and negative self-esteem on the part of people with disabilities. In other words, we continue to look at the vessel as half empty rather than half full. We all have weaknesses and limitations, but we also have strengths and abilities. Focusing on our strengths and abilities allows the joy of confidence and worth to be manifested in our self-concepts.

In our life experiences we acquire patterns of behavior based on our attitudes and beliefs. As we grow and mature these experiences help us become more competent in our functioning as human beings. We learn to understand the relationship between our wants and needs and we seek life experiences to satisfy our desires. The domains discussed above reflect our individuality, and our behavior is then expressed to those around us and the society as a whole.

Integrating our individual characteristics helps us to understand ourselves as we seek to change ineffective patterns of behavior. Personal growth and development occur as we begin to look inside ourselves and become aware of our whole beings. With this awareness comes the responsibility of making conscious choices and responding to others and our self with a clearer picture of who we really are. When these qualities of human life are expressed and shared with others, then life can be appreciated.

The traditional perspective of human development, as applied to disabled individuals, has served more to hinder the process of awareness and change. This can be attributed to the negative attitude held by many regarding disabilities. When we see a whole human being, a freeing process occurs and we see individuals with disabilities as people who happen to be on a different point of a continuum of human characteristics.

DISABILITY: A VARIATION
IN THE HUMAN CONDITION

Traditionally, disabilities are seen as abnormal conditions—deviations from the norm. Because we live in a world of social norms, people are constantly compared, studied, and evaluated according to established norms of human development and behavior. Anyone who deviates from that which is considered "normal" is often labeled, rejected, and isolated.

In many human-service fields, professionals now use the word *normal* with extreme caution. This new awareness can be attributed somewhat to the many social movements that have swept over society. People who are different in one way or another are asserting their rights and demanding access to the mainstream of society. Perhaps the liberation of any group of individuals is really the liberation of all people—the acceptance of diversity and variation in the human condition.

Disabilities can be viewed simply as natural variations in the human condition. This perspective is directly related to the ideology of *prosthetization*. Laird Heal explains this ideology in such a way that it not only views disabilities as variations in the human condition, but also stresses that they are normal and accepted variations. The author states:

> Prosthetization is the provision of prosthetic devices, such as eyeglasses and crutches, to handicapped individuals in order to facilitate their seeking integration into the larger society. . . . Compensation, by segregation, compounds the handicap by communicating to society and to handicapped individuals that unless they improve, they are unfit to participate in the society at large. Prosthetization, on the other hand, communicates that handicapped individuals are expected to participate in the larger society, and furthermore, promotes the development of intimate interactions among all citizens so that handicaps are seen to be common variations in the human condition rather than pitiful or repulsive pathologies.[3]

The acceptance of disabilities as variations in the human condition is an extremely positive and optimistic view of human beings. This ideology, when applied to service provision, allows therapeutic recreation specialists to view disabilities not as limitations but as variations in human behavior and ability. A positive and optimistic focus on a person's existing ability level will result in programs that build on strengths to increase human potential. Incorporating this ideology into our services will stimulate the elimination of programs that perpetuate the belief that disabilities are abnormal weaknesses that need to be remediated before people who possess them can "fit in" to society.

SIMILARITIES AND DIFFERENCES

People are mixtures of personal attributes and characteristics. These qualities that distinguish human beings from one another are diverse in nature. This diversity is a natural dimension of life and confirms the uniqueness that is endowed upon every individual. Strengths/weaknesses, abilities/disabilities, success/failures—all are dichotomies of the human experience.

The unique nature of every individual is generally thought to be a positive expression. However, the emphasis placed on unique and unusual traits can become so overwhelming that the similarities shared by all people are ignored. Failing to recognize that all individuals have the same basic human needs sets us apart from one another. This preoccupation with differences between people can place barriers to interpersonal relationships. Once these barriers become permanent structures, then the unique nature of human beings is lost and becomes a negative rather than a positive expression.

MOVEMENT TOWARD SELF-GROWTH

Human development is recognized and often described as a process through which human needs are satisfied. This theory has been espoused by Maslow; he describes a hierarchical structure containing five basic human needs: physiological needs, safety needs, belongingness and love needs, esteem needs, and self-actualization needs.[4] People who seek to satisfy their needs are also striving to realize their full human potential.

The fact that all people are developing as they meet their human needs helps us realize that disabling conditions which often separate people from one another are superficial characteristics with little relevance. We are alike in more ways than we are different. We share the joys of success and burdens of failure as we strive to satisfy our needs. The fact that we attempt to meet our needs in different ways is what makes all of us unique and special human beings.

As individuals with disabilities seek to satisfy their basic human needs (like any other person), they are confronted with four basic factors of human behavior that may affect their ability to satisfy their needs and ultimately realize their full potential. These four factors can be categorized as either positive or negative orientations to life's experiences and challenges. Figure 4-1 describes these factors and indicates the possible outcome these orientations may have on an individual's development.

The factors set forth in Figure 4-1 emphasize the basic difference between a positive and negative orientation to life. Granted, these represent two extreme views of human behavior, but they are presented in order to illustrate several major considerations that need to be recognized when working with individuals with disabilities.

Individuals' strengths, weaknesses, and the intensities of commitment to satisfy their needs varies with each person. Generalization about people's abilities and potentials for self-growth should not be based on any singular human characteristic (sex, race, ability, disability, or other social grouping). When generalizations are made they are usually based on stereotypes and/ or beliefs about one group of people or another.

Like other minority groups, people with disabilities have often been the victims of stereotypes and generalizations. As a result, many people have

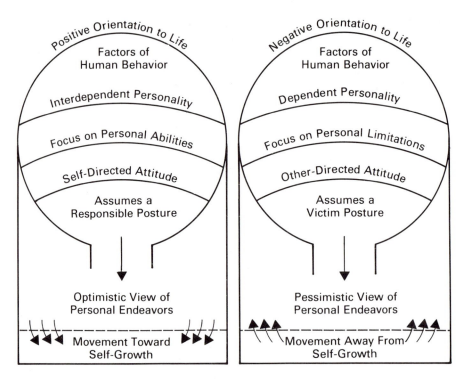

FIGURE 4-1 Life Orientation and Factors of Human Behavior

developed a pessimistic orientation to their personal lives and been subjected to a devalued position in society. Disabilities are only one characteristic of individuals and do not need to affect every aspect of their personalities; a full continuum of abilities and intensity of need is part of every individual's total personality and life structure. This understanding of human development must be applied in all helping professions if we are to enable people to satisfy their needs and realize their full potential.

FOCUS ON ABILITY

The importance of being aware of an individual's disabling condition when providing recreation services has been well documented. The issues of safety, liability, remediation, assessment, and skill development, to name a few, provide the therapeutic recreation specialist with evidence that suggests that the disabilities that participants possess dictate the types of programs and services they need and should receive. However, a word of caution should be applied to any therapeutic recreation specialist who provides services based on the disabling conditions possessed by program participants. This traditional approach to service delivery places too much emphasis on the disability and little or no regard to an individual's interest, human needs, or abilities. Frye and Peters note:

> Perhaps one of the most unfortunate effects of illness and disabilities is the tendency to group persons by their diagnosis, disability, or degree of mobility. Such grouping is often made for purposes of efficiency in treatment, but social grouping done along these lines is often inappropriate, ineffective, and artificial. Other than a common physical ailment, the people so grouped may have no other mutual interest on which to base a social relationship.[5]

Many benefits are afforded to the therapeutic recreation specialist who focuses on the abilities of a person with a disabling condition. These benefits, which have a direct effect on the quality of services provided, are listed below:

1. The leader is able to perceive an individual with a disability as a whole, developing human being.
2. The leader is able to recognize that people with disabilities are like any other human being in the most important ways.
3. The leader is able to develop problem-solving techniques to include people with disabilities in leisure experiences with their nondisabled peers.
4. The leader is able to plan leisure services for participants based on their interests and human needs.
5. The leader is able to design programs that encourage participants to become more independent and thus reduce their learned dependency on professionals.
6. The leader is able to design program environments that facilitate integration rather than segregation.
7. The leader is able to design situations in leisure programs that ensure the quality of social contact between disabled and nondisabled participants that may lead to a positive impact on their attitudes.
8. The leader is able to give up unnecessary control over people with disabilities and enable them to overcome their learned helplessness.
9. The leader is able to recognize disabled persons' skills, abilities, and unique talents and therefore learn from and work with them in a joint effort in planning programs to address needs.

SUMMARY

The primary focus of this chapter was to present a balanced perspective of persons with disabilities. Throughout this chapter we have been encouraged to move away from a traditional view of disabilities as abnormalities to appreciating disabilities as natural variations of the human condition. We have been challenged to get our lens in focus and center on the whole person. Once we begin to recognize the basic human needs we all share and to understand the differences we demonstrate in satisfying those needs, we will be able to move into a broader, more accepting understanding of what it means to be human.

Recreation professionals who embrace a balanced perspective regarding people with disabilities and believe in an optimistic orientation to their development are faced with the challenge of providing leisure services that reflect these values. This approach is not an easy one to apply. Once service providers can focus on the strengths of individuals with disabilities more than their weaknesses, then programs can be provided that will enable people with disabilities to assume greater responsibility and control over their own lives.

DISCUSSION QUESTIONS

4-1. List your personal characteristics in such areas as appearance, physical and mental ability, and social involvement. Think of these qualities as being on a continuum where at one end is society's "perfect" image and at the other end society's "imperfect" image. Place yourself on this continuum for each characteristic. Ask a friend, parent, or relative to do the same thing based on that person's perception of you. Compare and discuss the results. The following questions may help with the discussion.
   a. How were the continua alike or different?
   b. Did you learn anything new about how you perceive yourself or how others perceive you?
   c. How would you feel if people judged your whole personality based on one singular characteristic or society's projected image?

4-2. Refer to Figure 4-1 in the chapter. Think of two situations in your life experience, one positive, one negative. Reflect back on these experiences and think about your level of independence, ability to handle the situation, and your attitude toward it. How did you feel about yourself in both instances? What did you learn about your behavior in terms of your own personal growth?

4-3. What is the difference between a "segmented perspective" and a "balanced perspective" toward persons with disabilities?

4-4. What factors affect our personal "viewfinders" (our perceptions) toward persons with disabilities?

4-5. What are some benefits to focusing on abilities instead of disabilities?

4-6. How are disabilities similar to or different from other variations in the human condition?

4-7. What can you do to help yourself and/or others maintain a balanced perspective toward persons with disabilities?

NOTES

1. "Credo, Abilities" (New York: Human Resources Center, Inc., n.d.)

2. Clara Shaw Schuster and Shirley Smith Ashburn, *The Process of Human Development: A Holistic Approach* (Boston: Little, Brown, 1980), p. 23.

3. Laird W. Heal, "Ideological Responses of Society to its Handicapped Citizens," in *Integration of Developmentally Disabled Individuals into the Community*, eds. Anjela R. Novak and Laird W. Heal (Baltimore: Paul H. Brookes, 1980), pp. 39–40.

4. A. H. Maslow, *Motivation and Personality* (New York: Harper & Row, 1970), pp. 35–47.

5. Virginia Frye and Martha Peters, *Therapeutic Recreation: Its Theory, Philosophy, and Practice* (Harrisburg Penn.: Stackpole Books, 1972).

5

ATTITUDES TOWARD INDIVIDUALS WITH DISABILITIES

Sometimes negative stereotypes based on imagination or myths can cloud a person's perception of other human beings. This is an understandable phenomenon, but it does not have to be prolonged into lifelong attitudes. People's attitudes toward the handicapped can be changed by obtaining accurate information and experiencing positive encounters.[1]

INTRODUCTION

This chapter presents specific information on the nature of attitudes, myths, and stereotypes of disabilities and other factors that affect positive social interaction between disabled and nondisabled people. In addition, we will discuss the process and techniques for attitude change. It is hoped that this material will be personalized. That is, by relating this information to our own personal lives we will begin to understand the impact our positive and negative attitudes can have on our interpersonal relationships and our own personal growth.

FIGHT HANDICAPISM

An increase in awareness of societal prejudice toward disabled people is a direct result of the activism of the disability rights movement. The struggle to eliminate discriminating images of third world people, multicultural and ethnic groups, older people, and women has helped us become familiar with the concepts of racism, sexism, and agism. We can see practices of discrimination in many forms, reinforced in the literature and media and present in our social interaction patterns. We are all more aware or certainly becoming more aware of these practices and the need to work for their elimination. *Handicapism* refers to the attitudes and practices that lead to unequal and unjust treatment of people with disabilities.

Douglas Biklen and Robert Bogdan have studied the stereotypes regarding disabilities and have compared the similarities of racism, sexism, and agism to handicapism. The authors define handicapism as

> a theory and set of practices that promote unequal and unjust treatment of people because of apparent or assumed physical or mental disability. It manifests itself in relations between individuals, in social policy and cultural norms, and in the helping professions as well. Handicapism pervades our lives, but the concept of handicapism can also serve as a vital tool by which anyone can scrupulously examine personal and societal disabilities.[2]

Terminology

The word "handicap" originated from a game in which forfeits were drawn from a cap or hat. It is also linked with the practice of beggars who held "cap-in-hand" to solicit charity. This image certainly reflects the dependent position in which society placed disabled people.[3]

The language that is used to identify disabled people frequently reinforces society's misconceptions. Continued use of these terms perpetuates handicapism. The editors of *Bulletin:Interracial Books for Children* suggest preferred terms when making any necessary reference to disabled people. Table 5–1 describes these terms.

TABLE 5–1   Disability—Yes: Handicapped—No: The Language of Disability

OFFENSIVE	PREFERRED
handicap, handicapped person	disabililty, disabled person
deaf and dumb, deaf-mute, the deaf	deaf, hearing disability, hearing impairment
mongoloid	Down's syndrome
cripple, crippled	orthopedic disability, mobility impaired, disabled person
the blind	blind person, sight disability, visually impaired
retard, retardate, idiot, imbecile, feebleminded	retarded, mental impairment, mentally disabled
crazy, maniac, insane, mentally ill	emotional disability, emotional impairment, developmentally disabled

Related terms to avoid: The Minnesota 1976 Governors Conference on Handicapped Individuals proposed that the following entries be deleted from library catalogs: Abnormal children; Abnormalities, human; Atypical children; Children, backward; Children, retarded; Children, feebleminded.[4]

The specific terms outlined in Table 5-1 may vary in different geographical locations. Seeking the assistance of disabled consumers in the community to identify preferred terminology is an effective strategy. The process of labeling is a controversial issue and needs to be approached with sensitivity. There are some general guidelines to keep in mind that directly relate to our attitudes about labeling. These guidelines were developed by Target Access, a grant project at San Jose State University in California. They are designed to help service providers use appropriate language and terminology.

1. *Avoid Using Labels as Nouns*

   A label only describes one characteristic of an individual; therefore, use terms such as "a person with a hearing impairment, not "the deaf." When labels are used as nouns, e.g., emotionally disturbed, it tends to imply that all people with emotional problems are the same. Individuality is negated.

2. *Use Everyday Language*

   Using everyday language is acceptable with individuals with disabilities. For example, it is appropriate to use phrases such as "Did you see that movie on TV?" "Did you hear the news about . . . " "Would you like to go for a walk with me?"

3. *Attitudes and the Use of Labels*

   When the foundation of service providers' attitudes is based on equality and respect for all participants, then the language we use will reflect this attitude. However, sometimes we all make mistakes and use labels inappropriately. When this occurs, participants will understand that the intent is not rooted in negative attitudes. A sensitive leader may be open to learning from participants' suggestions.

4. *Negative Terms Perpetuate Myths*

   Avoid terms that depict the person as dependent or pitied and that perpetuate myths. For example: crippled, deaf-mute, retardate, idiot, insane.

5. *Avoid Using Labels*

   Describe the specific characteristic instead of using a disability label. "Mary has a difficulty comprehending what she reads" instead of "Mary has a learning disability." The latter statement is vague, accentuates differences, and may isolate Mary from her peer group. Think of a disability as just another characteristic in the spectrum of human differences that helps to make each person unique. Try using the phrase "people with varying abilities" instead of labels.[5]

The use of positive terms in our language, literature, and the media is one way to fight handicapism. Other strategies relate to attitude change, which will be discussed later in this chapter. In a speech eloquently delivered by Barbara Schneiderman, then director of the organization You, Me and Us (curriculum development of materials on disabilities), she described handicapism and suggested strategies for its elimination. Her speech is presented here for the reader's personal reflection.

Handicapism—What is it? It is a nondiscriminatory minority group. It is democracy in its purest form.

It has no respect for *classism.* Its membership represents all classes. Socioeconomic status, education, and training cannot buy you in or move you out of this minority group. Once you are a member, the membership can be lifetime.

It has no place within its ranks for *sexism.* It does not choose one sex over the other. Both sexes are equally represented.

It does not acknowledge *racism.* It does not discriminate among races. Being a member of a cultural or religious group neither guarantees your membership nor your exclusion.

It enrolls its members along a life continuum from birth to death. You do not find *agism* here.

Handicapism is a minority group with an open membership. Any one of us can become a member at any time, although we may not be able to choose our initiation day.

What do you get when you join this perfect nondiscriminatory democracy?

Well, first you get a big *label pin* which is given to you not by the members of the group but by the nonmembers.

Second, you get a printed set of instructions that remind you to wear your label pin at all major public and community events. Without your label pin, the nonmembers might not be able to differentiate you from "their" (nonmember) group. Wearing your label pin, you're told, protects you from the nonwearers for the nonwearers might just otherwise have unfair expectations of you and your capabilities.

Third, you get a hand-lettered wall motto that says "you are excused from participating in the majority group." You cannot. . . . You are not expected to. . . . You won't be able to. . . .

Fourth, you receive a leather-bound copy of a best seller entitled "Special Programs and Places for You," which includes listing of "special" education opportunities, "special" recreation services, "special" vocational training and "special" employment placement opportunities. You find the forward of your book never explains why "separate" is equated or synonymous with "special."

Fifth, you are given a self-teaching, self-correcting, self-reinforcing programmed instructional manual entitled "The New You—How To Develop An Adapted Identity."

The lessons provide instructions on how to change your feelings, your dreams, your ambitions.

You soon discover that you are to change or adapt your identity to meet the stereotyped attitudes of the majority group. Because they cannot see your sameness, only your difference. *You are to adapt your identity not so much to fulfill your needs as to fulfill the perceptions of others.*

Handicapism! The one true democracy? Maybe? Nonracist, Nonclassist, Nonagist. It almost sounds too perfect to be true.

But my only question to you: "Would you want to wear the label pin?"

The above may appear a little harsh. It was meant to be. For handicapism is a minority group one does not select but is selected for.

It is often easiest for those of us to understand what having to wear the handicapped label means if we can ask ourselves if we would want to wear the label.

If the answer is no, then we must work to dispense with the label, which is within our abilities to do as humans; for it is not always within our human abilities to control or change the membership of the group.

How do we go about throwing out the label?

First, we must begin to accept our own differences. Then we are on our way to accepting differences in others.

Second, we need to look at our attitudes. As a majority group are they based on fact or fiction? Do we perceive and relate to handicapped individuals as people first, and handicapped second, or as handicapped first and people second?

Third, we need to learn together, play together, work together, and do a whole lot of laughing and crying together. We must become willing to open ourselves to self-discovery and "other" people discovery.

Maybe, just maybe, if we could each commit to wearing one same label called "Humanism" all the other label "isms" would die—

Once and for all, and we could all be members of the same majority.[6]

SOCIETY'S DEVALUATION OF INDIVIDUALS WITH DISABILITIES

Individuals with disabilities have been devalued not only in American society but in many other cultures throughout the world. This painful reality has been frequently addressed and confirmed by research findings in the literature of education, psychology, sociology, anthropology, and recreation. This process of devaluation is related to the concept of *deviancy*, which has been studied by social scientists. Likewise, people with disabilities have also been perceived as deviant.

Adequately understanding the meaning of the terms *devalued* and *deviant* requires a careful examination of the word *value*. When something or someone has value, it is an accepted belief that the object or person is desirable and worthy of esteem—that the object or person is of quality and has intrinsic worth. There are many interpretations of the concept of deviancy in terms of the populations and behaviors that characterize this concept. Wolfensberger provides a definition of the concept of deviancy that takes into account its connection with the word *value*. The author states:

> a person can be said to be deviant if he is perceived as being significantly different from others in some aspect that is considered of relative importance, and if this difference is negatively valued.[7]

One of the premises of this chapter is the presumption that attitudinal barriers exist within society. Attitudes of nondisabled people toward disabled people have been the subject of many research studies. As we examine the concepts of value and deviancy we notice an interrelationship between the two. As we experience different facets of life we begin to recognize quite clearly the things in the world that society tends to value: money, power, beauty, productivity, and to a certain extent sameness. Historically, disabled people have not possessed these external "objects"; thus, internal qualities are often ignored because of attitudinal barriers.

In a study by Jerome Siller and colleagues in the Department of Educational Psychology at New York University, the existence of pervasive attitudinal barriers received substantial confirmation.

The researchers found six stable factors describing attitudes of nondisabled people toward individuals with disabilities. The disabilities explored were amputation, blindness, cosmetic conditions, deafness, obesity, and disability in general. These six factors are presented below:

> *Interaction Strain*—uneasiness in the presence of people with disabilities and uncertainty as to how to deal with them.
> *Rejection of Intimacy*—a rejection of close, especially intimate, relationships.
> *Authoritarian Virtuousness*—ostensibly "prodisabled," this orientation is rooted in an authoritarian context and advocates special treatment. Despite its benevolent appearance, the evidence suggests that it is fundamentally negative.
> *Inferred Emotional Consequences*—an assumption that disability impairs the character and emotions of its "victims."
> *Distressed Identification*—personalized reactions to disability arising from anxiety about one's own vulnerability.
> *Imputed Functional Limitations*—restricted evaluations of the ability of people with disabilities to function in the environment.[8]

THE IMPACT OF MYTHS AND STEREOTYPES

Historically, attitudes of the general public toward disabling conditions have been predominately negative. These attitudes have been primarily based on myths and stereotypes of disabilities. Uncertain or rejective perceptions of disabled people is a general reflection of society's lack of understanding of and sensitivity toward disabilities. This situation could easily be remedied if we were dealing only with people who needed and/or desired accurate information about conditions of impairment. Unfortunately, what has occurred in our society is that the general public has also acquired negative beliefs about the capabilities, personality characteristics, and potentials of people with disabilities solely on the basis of their rejective attitudes of the disabling condition. Tollifson, a disability rights activist, comments on the stereotypes of disabled people. She observes:

> Common stereotypes about disabled people are that we are weak, passive, incapable, overly sensitive, childlike, easily hurt, unable to make decisions, fragile, nonsexual and in need of protection. [People] should be made aware of the fact that we are not fragile. We won't break if we get bumped—in fact, we are strong and tough from surviving in a hostile world all our lives. Disabled people should be pictured as active, capable, physically strong, emotionally strong, able to run their own lives, sexual, etc.[9]

The personal acceptance and the perpetuation of the myths and stereotypes of disabled people represent a generalized pattern of societal response toward deviance. These patterns of negative beliefs have become attitudinal barriers that have not only prevented positive social interaction between disabled and nondisabled people but have also had a negative impact on the self-development of many individuals with disabilities.

> When a person is perceived as deviant he is cast into a role that carries with it powerful expectancies. Strangely enough, these expectancies not only take hold of the mind of the perceiver, but of the perceived person as well. It is a well-established fact that a person's behavior tends to be profoundly affected by the role expectations that are placed upon him. Generally, people will play the roles they have been assigned. This permits those who define social roles to make self-fulfilling prophecies by predicting that someone cast into a certain role will emit behavior consistent with that role. Unfortunately, role-appropriate behavior will then often be interpreted to be a person's "natural" mode of acting rather than a mode elicited by environmental events and circumstances.[10]

Society's negative response toward a disabling condition has subsequently resulted in the physical and social segregation of many human beings. People have been denied equal opportunities for achievement; their human behavior and personal expressions have been restricted. These limitations have produced a narrow range of role expectations. As a result, many people with disabilities have absorbed these stereotypes into their own self-concepts and have diminished their own aspirations.

Another consequence of society's attitude toward disability that has had a negative impact on people is the practice of labeling and categorizing. We often label objects as a way to identify and isolate those that require study and examination. This is usually done for practical and beneficial purposes. Unfortunately, the practice of labeling has gone beyond the disability itself and is used to describe human beings. The ways in which these labels are misused have greatly reduced the individuality of those who happen to have the disabling condition.

It is obvious that attitudes toward individuals with disabilities need to be changed. Some of the negative responses or attitudinal barriers that must be eliminated include:

1. The devaluation of disabled people solely on the basis of their disabling condition.
2. The labeling and classification practices of disabled people as deviant human beings.
3. The acceptance and perpetuation of myths and stereotypes of disabilities.
4. The prevention of social interaction between disabled and nondisabled people based on generalized negative beliefs.
5. The limited role expectations of people based on attitudes toward their disabilities and human characteristics.
6. The segregation of people with disabilities.
7. The lowered self-concept and diminished fulfillment of personal aspirations on the part of some people with disabilities.

PUBLIC ATTITUDES TOWARD DISABLED PEOPLE

Attitudes of the general public toward individuals with disabilities vary greatly. Social norms, values, personal experiences, and beliefs are influential in the formation of attitudes. Over the past several decades research studies have been conducted to analyze these attitudes, and although the results of these studies are not always consistent, Harold Yuker has summarized these findings as follows:

1. Although people make distinctions among types of disabilities, they also are willing to express attitudes toward disabled people in general. Even though individuals differ in the specific groups that they include when they speak of "handicapped," their attitudes toward people with different handicaps tend to be quite similar.
2. In response to direct questions, more than 50 percent of the people in the United States express slightly positive attitudes toward disabled people and indicate that they have sympathetic feelings for them. Other people, however, have negative, rejecting attitudes, and a few of them express these attitudes quite openly.
3. Many nondisabled individuals perceive handicapped people as "different" and in some ways inferior to "normal" people. They are uncomfortable in the presence of handicapped people. They "don't know how to behave," which implies that they believe one should behave differently in the presence of a person with a disability.
4. Despite the positive attitudes that are expressed in public, handicapped persons are often discriminated against. Many people favor segregation rather than integration of handicapped individuals. Possibly because of feelings that they are different, disabled people are often treated as if they were different.
5. Attitudes toward handicapped people often have negative aspects, the strength of which varies from one person to another. One such aspect relates to fears that "this could happen to me." Another relates to the tendency to reject people who are different.
6. Individual differences in attitudes are very large as a result of differences in people's knowledge and past experiences.[11]

THE NATURE OF ATTITUDES

Before examining our personal attitudes toward individuals with disabilities, let us first explore the nature of attitudes. The concept of *attitude*, which is somewhat confusing and ambiguous, has been a major focus of study in social psychology. It is a concept that is applied by many individuals, organizations, institutions, and researchers to interpret and explain diverse social and psychological phenomena. Social psychologists have defined attitude as a concept and a theory.

Definition of an Attitude

According to Fishbein and Ajzen, most social scientists would agree that

> An attitude can be described as a learned predisposition to respond in a consistently favorable or unfavorable manner with respect to a given object. It should be clear that since a person's attitude is assumed to be related to the total affect associated with his beliefs, intentions, and behaviors, we define response consistency in terms of overall evaluative consistency. Thus attitude is viewed as a general predisposition that does not predispose the person to perform any specific behavior. Rather, it leads to a set of intentions that indicate a certain amount of affect toward the object in question. Each of these intentions is related to a specific behavior, and thus the overall affect expressed by the pattern of a person's actions with respect to the object also corresponds to his attitude toward the object.[12]

This definition, like other interpretations, contains two key principles. First, attitudes are *learned* predispositions with the intent to respond in a positive or negative manner toward a person or object. Second, attitudes are composed of three components: a belief (cognitive) component, an emotional (affective) component, and an action (behavioral) component.[13] Attitudes are formed based on what we learn from significant people in our lives, personal experiences, and the media.

Attitudes and Behavior: Personal and Situational Influence

The relationship between attitudes and behavior is somewhat weak and conflicting. We have determined that behavior is one of the components of attitude. Behavior is defined as an "observable act taken by an individual in a specific situation."[14] Suggesting that our attitudes determine our behavior should be evaluated with caution, for there is not always a direct correlation between our beliefs and feelings about a person or object and our behavior toward that person or object.

Why is there such an inconsistent and nonsupportive relationship between attitude and behavior? It would seem that this relationship is vital to the development of community education programs to change the general public's attitudes toward individuals with disabilities. There must be factors that influence the expression of attitudes or the action taken. What are these social factors that may prevent individuals from acting in accordance with their convictions?

Researchers have concluded that interactional concepts such as norms, cultural values, reference groups, and subcultures influence the relationship between attitude and behavior.[15] Other social scientists suggest that social environmental factors such as the extent of social involvement, the number of social constraints, and the amount of peer pressure encountered by individuals may influence their behavior. As a result they do not act according to their attitude.[16]

PERSONAL ATTITUDES TOWARD DISABILITY

When we perceive an individual with a disability as "different," that person can experience stigma and personal stress. Likewise, we can experience a strain in our interactions with the disabled person and experience fears, personal stress, and avoidance. These are only a few of the many reactions that both groups face. Thus, it is important that we examine our attitudes toward disability in order to understand our social interaction patterns. The more we become aware of our belief systems and the accuracy upon which they are based, the greater our ability will be to facilitate positive interaction between disabled and nondisabled people.

Why Should We Examine Our Personal Attitudes?

As we have discussed, our attitudes are learned. If we choose, we can learn new concepts and change our attitudes. If we want others to become more accepting of differences, we need to be willing first to examine our attitudes and work to change them if necessary. People often attribute their behavior to environmental causes rather than personal factors. Examining personal attitudes may allow us to reflect on our own abilities to change our behavior. A willingness to look inward and examine our attitudes and their roots enables us to be open to change. Specific reasons for examining our attitudes are listed below. The reader is encouraged to consider each factor and to reflect upon his or her personal value and belief system and professional goals.

1. The therapeutic recreation professional is often considered a role model for participants and therefore has an influence on the participants' attitudes.[17]
2. While research on attitude change remains controversial, the literature suggests that a person in authority is in a position to effect attitude change.[18]
3. Individuals tend to act the way others perceive them. This phenomenon is generally referred to as the "Self-fullfilling Prophecy." This concept is critical since recreation personnel are in the business of facilitating growth and development. If a leader perceives and treats people with disabilities as helpless or devalues them, then they may begin to think of themselves in those terms.[19]
4. In order to develop empathy and respect for participants, leaders must examine their attitudes toward participants with disabilities. Effective interpersonal relationships are linked to an open, honest approach to people and the ability to feel comfortable with others.[20]
5. An awareness of personal and societal attitudes may give the leader an insight into one's own and others' behavior. Such insight can be valuable in resolving

conflict. Awareness of the effects of personal attitudes on the behavior and expectations of others can create a desire to change.[21]

6. Accepting a position as a professional carries with it a responsibility to promote the growth and development of human beings—that is, to make our influence positive and supportive.[22]

7. Paternalistic feelings and practices among professionals may develop if professionals perceive disabled individuals as subordinate and/or helpless.[23]

8. Professionals will be more inclined to answer children's questions and address parental concerns with ease and comfort if they have positive attitudes toward disabled people.

9. Negative stereotypes based on imagination or myths can cloud a person's perception of another human being.[24]

10. Examining personal attitudes will enable professionals to evaluate their level of expertise and knowledge about disabling conditions.

EXCLUSION: DEFINITION AND IMPACT

Perhaps at one time or another we have all experienced the feeling of being left out, ignored, "put down." The social situations, personal characteristics, or the circumstances that may have caused us to be excluded from human interaction are just as numerous as our responses to these negative experiences. As we look back and reflect upon some of these past experiences, it is safe to assume that we were probably questioning our personal identity and self-confidence. As a result, we may have been able only to react to the situation of being excluded from interacting with other people rather than being able to take control of the situation and assert ourselves. Our reaction to these experiences was probably evident in our negative feelings about ourselves, the situation, and the other participants.

People with disabilities, like any other human beings, have also felt the pains of exclusion. However, they often are excluded from social experiences solely on the basis of their disability. People who do not have to cope with a major disabling condition perhaps experienced the phenomenon of exclusion because they were fat, or wore braces, or couldn't catch a baseball! But in both instances, people are often excluded from participating in many social experiences solely on the basis of a single human characteristic.

The phenomenon of exclusion has been defined as "a barring of the Other from oneself, a disregarding of the Other as a human presence in a face-to-face situation."[25] Understanding the term *exclusion* requires a deeper examination of the impact this phenomenon may have on an individual. Geller, Goodstein, Silver, and Sternberg, who have studied the effects of being ignored, provide a definition of exclusion that describes not only its effect on people but also the correlation that exists between being ignored and subsequent interpersonal relationships. The authors report:

> To be ignored is to be excluded while physically present. One's opinions are unsolicited, comments unwanted, approval unneeded. It is the violation of the expectations built up in daily social intercourse. In the extreme, being ignored is a form of powerlessness. It means that a person cannot exert social control over the situation. One's attention or lack of attention, leaving or staying will make no difference; one's comments are unimportant as are one's reaction to the comments of others.
>
> Because of this powerlessness, the ignored person is not in a position to act, only react. . . .
>
> Since an ignored person is looked at and talked to infrequently, he will feel less liked and therefore like himself less than someone who has not been ignored. Similarly, ignored persons will have a less favorable impression of the persons ignoring them than they might have had in a normal situation. Since people perceive being ignored as a negative evaluation, it is not surprising that they will respond in kind.
>
> Although an ignored person may not retaliate overtly, subtle retaliations may be made if an opportunity develops. It would be expected that an ignored person, for example, would withhold a reward from someone who has ignored him.[26]

The negative consequences of exclusion not only hinder the quantity and quality of interpersonal relationships but also adversely affect an individual's self development.

> While feeling excluded and self-conscious, the individual is unable to live his or her immediate experience as a total, integrated person.[27]

This consequence can be devastating to any individual. But to the person with a disability, this lack of social acceptance perpetuates the emphases that are often placed on the disabling condition rather than the personality and humanness of the person. This may seem like an insignificant point, but its impact on the acceptance, respect, and inclusion of people with disabilities in social situations has been clearly documented throughout history.

Sources of Exclusion

The sources of exclusion are many and varied. According to Anderson, the main mechanism of exclusion is identified as "emotional distancing." Within this phenomenon there are two categories of descriptive behaviors; the attitudes or demeanor of the helper, and physical and verbal expressions. Even though these behaviors were observed within a health care system, the phenomenon itself can be observed in most social situations as well.[28]

In addition to an individual's attitudes of impatience, displeasure, authority, and physical and verbal expressions (facial, tone of voice, verbal style, use of silence, use of eyes, and use of touch) described by Anderson, there are many other ways in which people with disabilities are often excluded. Listed below are some examples of how individuals with disabilities are often excluded in recreation settings.

1. *Architectual barriers* (stairs, heavy doors, narrow doorways, and so forth) often found in recreation and park facilities prevent disabled people from having access not only to the building or park but also to the services.

2. *The use of negative terminology and labels* ("deaf and dumb," "retard," "crazy," "crippled") perpetuates myths and stereotypes of disabilities and accentuates differences.

3. *Segregated programs on the basis of disabling conditions* (rather than leisure interests) limit opportunities for disabled and nondisabled people to share leisure experiences and learn about one another.

4. *Inappropriate intervention or lack of intervention by the leader* can hinder the quantity and quality of social relationships developed between disabled and nondisabled participants.

5. *Parental concerns* or their lack of accurate information about disabilities may discourage integrated programs. Also parental overprotection on the part of parents of disabled children may perpetuate segregated programs.

6. *Inaccessible publicity and media relations* may exclude disabled people from knowing about community events and programs.

7. *Negative attitudes and fears* regarding disabling conditions may reduce social interaction between disabled and nondisabled people.

8. *Negative self-concepts and self-confidence* on the part of disabled people may reduce their desire to participate in programs with their nondisabled peers.

9. *Lack of social/leisure skills* of disabled people may prevent their inclusion in recreation programs with nondisabled people.

10. *Extensive "specialized services"* may discourage general recreation personnel from wanting to include disabled people in their programs.

Exclusion, Seclusion, and Inclusion

The total elimination of exclusion from all human interaction may not be possible, but examining the ways in which people with disabilities are excluded in recreation and leisure experiences and social relationships may stimulate therapeutic recreation personnel to modify their facilitation and intervention techniques. Developing an awareness of human-relations strategies will give the specialist the necessary tools to enable program participants to control their exclusion and the subsequent feelings associated with this negative aspect of socialization.

In order to help all program participants develop a realistic and effective method for taking control of their feelings associated with being excluded, it is important that participants fully understand the differences among exclusion, seclusion, and inclusion. Table 5–2 compares the social phenomena of exclusion, seclusion, and inclusion in terms of their definitions and impact upon people who may experience these occurrences in social situations.

By examining Table 5–2, it is easy to see that exclusion and inclusion are direct opposites of one another. The positive and negative consequences of these types of social situations can spell the difference between enabling individuals with disabilities to value and assert themselves or perpetuating the segregation of this group of people from their nondisabled peers.

TABLE 5-2 Exclusion, Seclusion, Inclusion: A Comparison

FACTORS	EXCLUSION	SECLUSION	INCLUSION
Definition	To ignore some-one's physical and social presence	To be left alone, but not left out; to maintain verification of the value of the person	To be accepted as part of a whole; to be contained and involved
Outcome/impact	Powerless, negative self-identity, withdrawal	Rest, privacy, relief from stress of interactional relationships	Positive self-identity, sense of control, self-respect, and concern for others
Associated feelings	Helplessness, anger, self-consciousness, "out-of-place," insignificant	Protected, secure, private	Accepted, embraced, confident, valued

Seclusion, on the other hand, is the boundary of exclusion. What is meant by this is that there exists a fine line between being left alone and left out. We all need time to be alone, to examine our different "selfs," if we are to grow and develop to our fullest potential. But as therapeutic recreation specialists we have the responsibility to confirm consistently the identity and existence of our program participants if we are to prevent seclusion (which implies rest and relief) from becoming exclusion.

There is a choice and a decision to be made in every human interaction. Participants are faced with these choices and decisions in their relationships with one another. We all have the potential to control the conditions governing human interactions and the environments in which they occur, both of which impact on ourselves and others. We can negate or confirm one another. In social situations between disabled and nondisabled individuals within our recreation programs, specialists have the responsibility to enable participants to support and accept one another. Thus, specific leadership techniques will be discussed throughout the text.

ATTITUDE CHANGE

As we have discussed, the relationship between attitude and behavior is vague and conflicting. The behavior component of an attitude is significant because that is what we hope to change when attempts are made to change attitudes. Much has been written about the negative beliefs and attitudes of the general public toward disabled people. However, the literature contains relatively few studies that clearly indicate intervention techniques that can be used to modify attitudes toward the disabled.[29] But there do exist some common factors to successful intervention strategies. This next section will review these factors and suggest some implications for the therapeutic recreation professional.

Educational Programs

Educational programs aimed at altering attitudes toward disabled people can include many different direct and indirect techniques to elicit the change. The design of the program will certainly depend on the strengths of the trainers, personal and situational factors that influence relationships, and behavior and learning opportunities. Because so many issues affect the design of a program, it is probably more important to understand the role of educational programs. Iverson and Portnoy discuss this role by showing the relationship among knowledge, attitudes, and behavior. They state:

> The assumed role of educational programs in behavior change is to directly increase knowledge and indirectly initiate attitude and behavior changes. Knowledge then functions as a direct and indirect stimulus for change in attitudes and a direct change agent for behavior. Knowledge will function as a direct change agent for attitudes far more frequently than it will for behaviors. Attitudes are direct and indirect change agents for behavior. Once a behavior is altered there is, in many instances, a direct feedback mechanism which alters the appropriate attitudes in such a manner as to reinforce the new behavior or reduce any dissonance.[30]

Educational and informational programs appear to result in a positive attitude change and increased acceptance of people with disabilities about 50 percent of the time. Yuker has synthesized the factors that seem to influence the effectiveness of the communication. These factors include:

1. The content of the message and the medium through which it is presented;
2. The source of the communication;
3. The characteristics of the person who receives the communication;
4. The behavior engaged in by the person who receives the communication.[31]

The process of attitude change is a complex one, but the factors cited above can serve as guidelines in developing educational programs. Knowledge of disability hierarchies may also be helpful and serve as a guideline for developing educational programs, because they relate to attitude change. Yuker summarizes society's level of acceptance of disabilities:

1. The most acceptable handicaps are those that are comparatively minor such as people who are partially seeing, speech handicapped, have heart disease or an ulcer, are hard of hearing, etc.;

2. Next most acceptable are people who have suffered the loss of one or more extremities such as persons who are paralyzed or amputees, etc;
3. The middle category consists of people with the complete loss of a major sense such as vision or hearing;
4. People who are mentally ill tend not to be accepted and are usually rejected;
5. People with acute and chronic brain injuries such as epilepsy, cerebral palsy, or mental retardation are at the bottom of the list of acceptability.[32]

This list is included only as an overview and should be used with extreme caution. This list does, however, relate to attitude change in that the attitudes associated with groups at the top of the list are easier to change than those at the bottom of the list.

Techniques for change. The techniques enumerated below can be used in changing attitudes toward individuals with disabilities. Any one of these methods if used alone will not be as effective as combining two or more of them. These techniques have been synthesized from the literature and include direct as well as indirect methods. It is important to remember that nothing will work with everyone or be effective all of the time because of the nature of attitudes coupled with the issues we have discussed throughout this chapter.

1. *Information Campaigns.* Multimedia communication presentations to a specific, carefully defined audience, with the public being asked to make a commitment to their new attitude.[33]
2. *Role-Playing.* Interaction between two people aimed at reversing roles (participant/leader, disabled participant/nondisabled participant, and so forth).[34]
3. *Counterattitudinal Advocacy.* Individuals required to prepare and give a speech or lecture advocating attitudes opposite their own.[35]
4. *Public Commitment.* People asked to make either a public statement of their point of view or their intention to do a specific thing (for example, make restaurant accessible to wheelchair users).
5. *Contact with or Exposure to Disabled Persons.* Structured opportunities for interaction between disabled and nondisabled persons of equal status and with disabled people who do not fit stereotyped roles and characteristics.
6. *Changing the Environment.* Eliminating barriers in the physical and social environment that prevent equal access for disabled people.
7. *Social Skill Development.* Opportunities for disabled people to develop appropriate social skills if necessary.
8. *Integrated, Cooperative Play Experiences.* Opportunities for disabled and nondisabled people to interact in cooperative (not competitive) play experiences (New Games, Movement Exploration Techniques and Approaches).
9. *Disability Simulations.* Structured opportunities for nondisabled people to simulate disabling conditions and observe reactions of nondisabled peers.[36]
10. *Puppetry.* Structured opportunities for children to manipulate "disabled" puppets or be an audience in a puppet show (for example, Kids on the Block, Inc.).[37]
11. *Human Differences Training.* Structured opportunities to recognize, understand, and deal with differences and similarities between people.[38]

12. *Professional Training.* Participation in professional training opportunities (in-service training conferences, workshops, educational courses, and so forth).[39]

13. *Contact and Educate Media.* Contact media resources (newspapers, magazines, radio and television, wire services, newsletters) and suggest guidelines for de-picting disabled people in positive roles.[40]

These techniques can all be modified to suit the unique variables of the community involved and its existing attitudes toward disabled people. In any effort to change attitudes, we should try to develop understanding and empathy regarding individuals with disabilities. Our primary goal is to in-crease options for all people and enhance our social interaction patterns and level of acceptance for human differences. Donaldson comments on two basic actions that can both result in positive attitude change. The author states:

> In summary, it appears that positive attitude change or reduced avoidance will result when an exposure to handicapped persons is powerful enough to change a presently held stereotype by either (a) significantly reducing discomfort, uneasiness, or uncertainty on the part of the nonhandicapped and/or (b) pre-senting enough information to contradict the presently held stereotype that the present attitude is "unfrozen" or changed.[41]

SUMMARY

In American society, the attitudes toward individuals with disabilities have historically been negative. Myths and stereotypes seem to characterize each disability, and subsequent generalizations are made about people who are labeled with some type of disability. Social prejudices toward disabled people are similar in nature to other devalued groups in our society.

Attitudes are learned predispositions and are composed of three parts: belief, emotion, and action. These components—when combined with norms, cultural values, reference groups, and subcultures—influence human behav-ior. Attitude-change strategies are directed at altering human behavior to al-low for the acceptance of individuals with disabilities and their increased integration into the mainstream of society.

Therapeutic recreation professionals who carefully examine their atti-tudes toward disability can act as powerful role models in the process of in-tegration. Personal awareness allows the professional to develop empathy and respect for individual differences.

DISCUSSION QUESTIONS

5–1. Why should we be careful with the language we use regarding persons with disabilities?

5–2. What is meant by a "self-fulfilling prophecy"?

5-3.   What are the three components that comprise attitudes?

5-4.   Identify four reasons we should examine our personal attitudes toward persons with disabilities.

5-5.   What are some ways that persons with disabilities may be excluded in recreation settings?

5-6.   Name and describe two techniques for changing attitudes.

NOTES

1. Ann P. Turnbull and Jane B. Schulz, *Mainstreaming Handicapped Students: A Guide for the Classroom Teacher* (Boston: Allyn & Bacon, 1979), pp. 341–342.

2. Douglas Biklen and Robert Bogdan, "Handicapism in America," *Win* (1976).

3. Douglas Biklen and Robert Bogdan, "Media Portrayals of Disabled People: A Study in Stereotypes," *Bulletin: Interracial Books for Children*, 8, no. 6–7 (1977), 4.

4. Ibid, p. 5.

5. Kathleen Collard, and others, *Closing the Gap: An In-service Training Guide for Mainstreaming Recreation and Leisure Services* (San Jose State University: Dept. of Recreation and Leisure Studies, 1980).

6. Barbara Schneiderman, "Handicapism." Speech presented at California Association for Physical Education, Health and Recreation Conference, March 1978.

7. Wolf Wolfensberger, *The Principle of Normalization in Human Services* (Toronto, Canada: National Institute of Mental Retardation, 1972), p. 13.

8. *Rehab.: Bringing Research Into Effective Focus.* Continuing Research Findings: Attitudes Toward People with Disabilities. National Institute of Special Education and Rehabilitation Services, Washington, D.C., Vol. 5, No. 10, (October 1982), 1–4.

9. Joan Tollifson, "An Open Letter," *Bulletin: Interracial Books for Children* 8, no. 6–7 (1977), 19.

10. Wolfensberger, *Principle of Normalization*, pp. 15–16.

11. Harold E. Yuker, "Attitudes of the General Public Toward Handicapped Individuals," *Awareness Papers* (Washington, D.C.: White House Conference on Handicapped Individuals, 1977), p. 94.

12. Martin Fishbein and Icek Ajzen, *Belief, Attitude, Intention and Behavior: An Introduction to Theory and Research* (Reading, Mass.: Addison-Wesley, 1975), p. 15.

13. Yuker, "Handicapped Individuals," p. 93.

14. Donald C. Iverson and Barry Portnoy, "Reassessment of the Knowledge/Attitude/Behavior Triad," *Health Education*, November/December, 1977, p. 32.

15. L. G. Warner and M. L. DeFleur, "Attitude as an Interactional Concept: Social Constraint and Social Distance as Intervening Variables Between Attitudes and Actions," *American Sociological Review*, 34 (1969), 153–169.

16. M. L. DeFleur and F. R. Westie, "Attitude as a Scientific Concept," *Social Forces*, 42 (1963), 17–31.

17. Collard and others, *Closing the Gap*, p. 16.

18. Ibid., p. 17.

19. Ibid.

20. Ibid., p. 18.

21. Ibid.

22. Robert F. Mager, *Developing Attitude Toward Learning* (Belmont, Calif.: Fearon-Pitman Publishers, 1968), p. 99.

23. John G. Schroedel, *Attitudes Toward Persons with Disabilities* (New York: Human Resources Center, A Project PREP Publication, 1979), p. 60.

24. Ann P. Turnbull and Jane B. Schulz, *Mainstreaming Handicapped Students: A Guide for the Classroom Teacher* (Boston: Allyn & Bacon, 1979), p. 34.

25. Nancy Anderson, "Exclusion: A Study of Depersonalization in Health Care," *Journal of Humanistic Psychology*, 21, No. 3 (1981), 67–68.

26. Daniel Geller, L. Goodstein, M. Silver, and W. Sternberg, "On Being Ignored: The Effects of the Violation of Implicit Rules of

Social Interaction," *Sociometry,* 37, No. 4 (1974), 541.

27. Anderson, "Exclusion," p. 73.

28. Ibid., pp. 71–72.

29. Joy Donaldson, "Changing Attitudes Toward Handicapped Persons: A Review and Analysis of Research," *Exceptional Children,* 46, No. 7 (April 1980), 505.

30. Iverson and Portnoy, "Reassessment," p. 33.

31. Yuker, "Attitudes of the General Public," p. 98.

32. Ibid., p. 97.

33. Ibid., p. 102.

34. Ibid., p. 103.

35. Ibid.

36. Donaldson, "Changing Attitudes," p. 508.

37. Barbara Aiello, "Hey, What's It Like to Be Handicapped?" *Education Unlimited,* 1, No. 2 (June 1979), 28–30.

38. Susan Stainback and William Stainback, "Educating Nonhandicapped Students: A Human Differences Training Model," *Education Unlimited,* 3, No. 2 (March/April 1981), 17–19.

39. Schroedel, *Persons with Disabilities,* p. 18.

40. *How to Make Friends and Influence the Media* (Falls Church, Va: Institute for Information Studies, 1979), pp. 10–16.

41. Donaldson, "Changing Attitudes," p. 510.

6

THE NATURE
OF DISABILITY
Social-Cultural, Environmental, and Psychological Factors

In spite of so many destructive attitudes and practices freely and openly practiced by society, psychologists, educators, and rehabilitation personnel, there are many disabled individuals who manage to survive the "system" and emerge as unique, proud human persons. Primarily they are those who are able to externalize their disability, and the attitudes toward it, as something put upon them which may cause certain limitations and with which they must contend. But they see this as only one aspect of themselves, representing only a small portion of what they really are—persons like all people and with all the wondrous possibilities of everyone else.[1]

INTRODUCTION

The primary concern of therapeutic recreation specialists is the provision of leisure services for individuals with disabilities. As service providers we are charged with the responsibility of developing a thorough understanding of the nature of disabling conditions. This base of knowledge, along with an understanding of the therapeutic recreation process of intervention, provides guidelines for the specialist to use in the coordination of services for individuals with disabilities.

Recent developments and changes in the methods of service delivery (that is, normalization, deinstitutionalization, integration, and mainstreaming) cause us to examine the level of knowledge regarding disabling conditions needed by professionals. A mere basic understanding of the characteristics and safety precautions of disabling conditions does not give the service provider an accurate picture of a "whole" human being. Service providers who choose to plan therapeutic recreation services that reflect the ecological perspective need to acquire an understanding of the social-cultural, environmental, and psychological aspects of disability. It is safe to assume that we have always needed this depth of understanding, but as our profession has evolved we have broadened our knowledge and can now see the interrelationships between the social sciences and therapeutic recreation. The use of social psychological theories and research, specifically as they relate to our understanding of disabling conditions, is essential to the process of therapeutic recreation intervention.

This chapter will discuss the major social-cultural, environmental, and psychological aspects of disability. The information is presented as an overview, but the material selected for inclusion in this chapter has the most relevance for therapeutic recreation specialists. The intent of this chapter, then, is to help us acquire a thorough understanding of the nature of disability.

ADJUSTMENT: COPING AND ADAPTATION

The causes of disabling conditions are diverse, complex, and sometimes unknown. The identified causes of disability include hereditary factors; complications that arise before, during, or after the birth process; infections or diseases; drugs, accidents, or trauma.

Regardless of the origin of the disability, we need to be aware of how the disability may impact on the individual's lifestyle.

> The age of onset may influence the person's acceptance of the disability as well as affect their development. In addition to the age of onset, the extent of the disability, the impact on the lifestyle, and the amount of personal and family acceptance each play an important role in the eventual adjustment and rehabilitation of the individual. Individual personality, experience and motivation also determine the extent to which people challenge themselves and maximize their potentials.[2]

Understanding the nature of disability begins by considering basic factors related to adjustment, for the process of coping with illness and disability involves certain biological, psychological, social, and environmental responses in order to deal with the condition adequately. Much has been written in rehabilitation literature regarding the importance of modifying biological and physical environments to the overall success of the rehabilitation process.

Several case studies were reviewed in preparing material for this chapter. The cases reviewed demonstrated that some contention exists among the degree of disability, physical and biological rehabilitation, environmental modification, and the successful psychological and social adaptation of the individual with the condition. There were just as many examples of people who successfully coped with and adapted to their disability, after a systematic process of rehabilitation, as there were those who had not achieved success.

What, then, are the factors that affect an individual's ability to cope with and adapt to his or her disability? Given the same process of rehabilitation, why do some people achieve success while others experience failure? Obviously biological and environmental conditions are important components in an individual's overall adjustment. But the social and psychological state of the individual must also be carefully considered.

Injury that results in permanent disability is often considered a crisis situation. This type of situation refers to an individual who is "confronted with adaptive tasks that demand the mobilization of new resources in psychological competence and social skills."[3] Coping comes into play when the individual has to develop strategies and a style for adapting to having a disability.

Coping psychologically to any kind or degree of disability with success necessitates a positive self-concept. Coping, in the context of this chapter, is not to be viewed as a pragmatic approach to human existence. Rather, it is a process that demands personal strength and determination. Calhoun and Acocella provide a perspective on adjustment as espoused by humanistic psychologists. The authors state:

> The humanists argue that ideal adjustment involves a great deal more than simply coping, or even coping happily, with the circumstances of your life. Rather, adjustment requires that the individual develop all her human capabilities to the fullest. It is not enough to meet one's basic needs for food, warmth, respect, and love; the individual must proceed beyond these satisfactions to the fulfillment of some ideal that is uniquely hers and generated only by herself. . . . If the individual's expectations for herself are narrow and rigid, she will have to deny large portions of her experience and spend all her energies defending her self-concept. But if she can meet life openly and accept her responses to experience, then she will achieve the ideal adjustment—that is, continued growth, based on a firm self-esteem.[4]

Another reason why the psychological state of the disabled person is crucial to his or her adaptation rests with society's lack of acceptance of anyone who deviates from the concepts of "body-whole" and "body-beautiful." Sometimes, no matter how hard individuals work on their rehabilitation, society continues to stigmatize them.

> The full restoration of function does not typically result in his acquisition of fully normal status. The change of status is from that of one with a defect to someone with a history of having corrected a defect, but the stigma of having

been defective still persists. The "reformed" alcoholic, the "cured" drug addict, and the ex-mental-patient are still perceived as more vulnerable and less-complete human beings than are individuals with no such histories of deviancy.[5]

Another social-psychological factor that aids an individual with a disability during their adjustment process is emotional or social support. As we reflect back on our own personal lives, we have all had experiences or crises in which we sought help and/or support from our families, friends, or a member of the helping profession. The emotional support we received perhaps helped us to cope with the situation and to adapt to personal changes in our lives. Disability can be one of those situations in which support can facilitate coping and adaptation.

What do we mean by *social (emotional) support?* How can social interactions help us to deal more effectively with stressful situations? Perhaps the best way to understand this phenomenon is to examine the definition of social support.

> Social support is defined as information leading the subject to believe that he is cared for and loved, esteemed, and a member of a network of mutual obligations. It appears that social support can protect people in crisis from a wide variety of pathological states: from low birth weight to death, from arthritis through tuberculosis to depression, alcoholism, and the social breakdown syndrome. Furthermore, social support may reduce the amount of medication required, accelerate recovery, and facilitate compliance with prescribed medical regimens.[6]

AN OVERVIEW OF FACTORS

The nature of disability is multifaceted. It involves a dynamic interrelationship among three major factors—social-cultural, environmental, and psychological. Specific elements of each factor will be presented in this chapter. An effective method for understanding the interrelationship of these factors is to examine a visual presentation. First, let us look at each factor individually, become familiar with its elements, and then view the whole model. Figure 6-1 illustrates the social-cultural factor. Figure 6-2 adds to the first with the addition of the environmental factor. Finally, Figure 6-3 illustrates all three factors.

Each of the specific elements of the three factors will be discussed. However, before the discussion begins, it would be helpful to review the model as a whole in order to see the interrelationship of the factors and the impact they may have on an individual's ability to adjust to the disability. Figure 6-4 shows the model in its entirety, and it includes the general factors discussed in the beginning of this chapter.

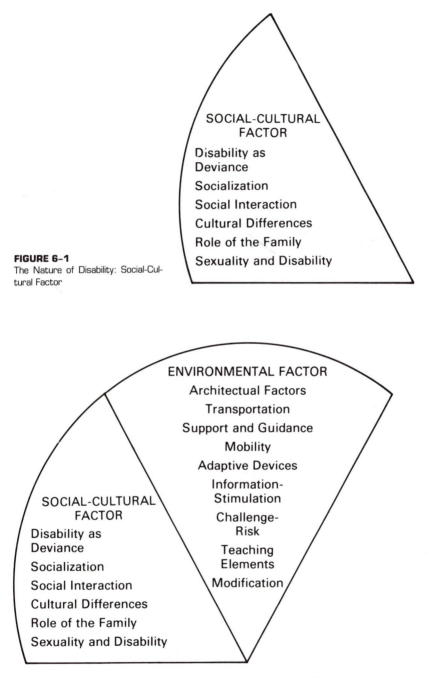

FIGURE 6-1
The Nature of Disability: Social-Cultural Factor

FIGURE 6-2   The Nature of Disability: Social-Cultural and Environmental Factors

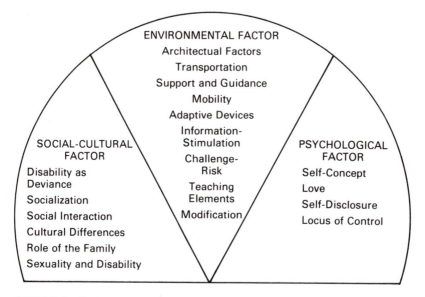

FIGURE 6-3   The Nature of Disability: Social-Cultural, Environmental, and Psychological Factors

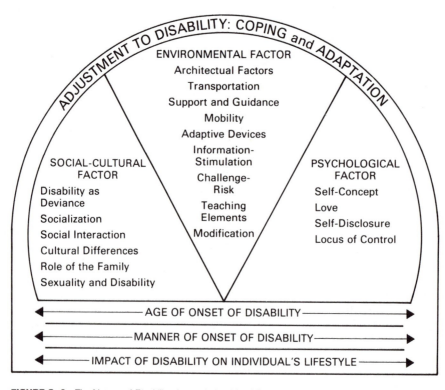

FIGURE 6-4   The Nature of Disability: Interrelationship of Factors

SOCIAL-CULTURAL FACTORS

Disability as Deviance

Ever since the 1940s, disability has been perceived and defined within the sociological context of *deviance*. Deviance is defined by many sociologists as "behavior that violates institutionalized expectations or behavior that represents departure from societal norms."[7] This perception and classification policy, which is often used to describe disabled people, implies that something is inherently "wrong" with the individual. This manner of viewing disabled people regards disability as a "social problem" similar to crime, drugs, prostitution, and delinquency. When disabilities are judged in this manner we are not able to perceive disabilities as variations of the human condition as discussed in Chapter 3.

As a result of this perception (disability as a social problem), society has assigned several deviant roles to disabled people. These historical social roles are listed below:

1. Sick Person
2. Subhuman Organism
3. Social Menace
4. Unspeakable Object of Dread
5. Object of Pity
6. Holy Innocent
7. Diseased Organism
8. Object of Ridicule
9. Eternal Child
10. Sinister and Evil
11. Curious Objects
12. Social Burden
13. Super Crip
14. Nonsexual

It is obvious that the above roles are not positive ones. They focus on the differences of disabled people, and the difference is believed to be negative. People who are placed in these roles by society, and who accept this perception about themselves, have the potential of living a limited, dependent existence. They may even be placed within environments that reflect these negative values.

The process of labeling is the result of society's reaction to deviance. Society responds to disability by labeling individuals, categorizing, and segregating them from the mainstream of society. Disabled people are often a population who are perceived as having little power and few resources; as a result, they are often placed in a category and labeled as such. The result of this process is that an individual's position in society is changed (low social status), and limited social roles are applied. Individuals who accept this position may diminish their self-concepts.

Constantina Safilios-Rothschild's perspective of disability as deviance further illuminates the impact of the process of labeling. The author observes:

> The disabled can best be analyzed and explained by means of the general theory of deviance. As with all other deviants, it is not so much their actual physical disability that is the key, but rather society's reaction to it. The disabled are not intrinsically deviant because of their disability, but because those around them label them "deviant" since they impute to them an undesirable difference. The resulting limitations render an individual more or less dependent and therefore deviant since he must break the norm of adult independence and self-reliance.[8]

The labels that are often placed upon people can be damaging and permanent. Often, predicted behavior accompanies a label. In the case of people with disabilities, these labels are generalized to all people in this minority group. Individuality is lost because society expects deviant behavior to be demonstrated by the labeled population.

> The literature of disability as deviance has argued that, like other stigmatized groups, the disabled tend to be evaluated as a category, rather than as individuals. The physical characteristic becomes a master trait, swamping personal differences.[9]

Labels are often assigned to people at a very early age. Kate Long comments on the labeling process as it is used in the public school system. She notes:

> If somebody calls you a turkey, a genius, or a creep, you've been labeled for that minute, sure enough. But even though a name can hurt as well as feel good, it's just an opinion and usually doesn't permanently affect your idea of who you are and what you can do. When a child in public school is officially labeled retarded, emotionally disturbed, brain damaged, or learning disabled, however, the label is regarded as a factual statement about the child. Because the weight of the school system's judgment is behind the label, it is hard for the child and those who know the child to disregard the label, particularly if it is used to segregate him or her from unlabeled classmates. Such labels often adhere to a person throughout life.[10]

It is obvious that labels often carry with them negative connotations. These labels have had a disturbing impression upon young children. Thurman and Lewis comment on this problem:

> Simply, it may be suggested that the roots of prejudice and rejection of handicapped children may lie in the tendency to respond differentially to difference. When labels with negative connotations are placed on these already discriminable differences, prejudices are likely to result.[11]

Socialization

The term *socialization* often refers to "the sequence of social learning experiences that result into a society."[12] This process involves interaction with family members, friends, groups of people, institutions, and the environment. Diverse relationships in a variety of settings help us to learn appropriate and acceptable behavior in human relationships. This diversity of experience is necessary because the process of socialization is long and complex.

Disabled people who have limited opportunities for social learning may experience difficulty in adjusting and fitting into society. Disabled people are often segregated from their nondisabled peers and as a result may not learn a full range of behavior but may model their behavior after the group with which they have the most contact. People who have been institutionalized may exhibit behavior that goes unnoticed in an institution but would be rejected in an integrated environment. Research indicates that in integrated settings, children imitate their nondisabled peers most frequently.[13] It appears that nondisabled children are more effective role models in helping disabled children learn appropriate social behavior.[14]

An aspect of social learning involves the opportunity to carry out different social roles. Social status or social position allows individuals to acquire basic skills and knowledge necessary to demonstrate responsible behavior. This aspect of social learning, as well as the whole process of socialization, can have an impact on the development of one's self-concept. Michael Teague suggests the following:

> It has long been asserted that mental health and illness are directly related to social-environmental conditions. Also, one may contend that self-concept depends partially on the way one performs in his everyday social positions and the way others react to him.[15]

Social Interaction

The social environment can significantly influence the quality of interaction between disabled and nondisabled people. The ability of disabled people to adjust successfully to their condition will depend on the interaction among their personality, the environment, and social variables. When maladjustment has occurred, sociologists and psychologists have often pondered as to the possibility of a "handicapped personality." However, research findings refute this concept. Leo Buscaglia, an educator who reports this research, provides an explanation for maladjustment that has special application to therapeutic recreators. The author states:

> So those with disabilities are simply people. The individuals become handicapped to the extent to which they internalize their limitations as debilitating and undesirable. Their attitudes will be largely determined by the labels im-

posed upon them, the society's reaction to these labels and the special treatment they receive. In addition, destructive, segregated environments and isolating behaviors which tend to remove them from the world will serve to convince them further of their handicaps. This is visibly enacted in many so-called "rehabilitation" programs whose main function seems to be to define and label handicaps, select those who fit their labels, segregate these individuals and help them conform to what the rehabilitators believe are the individual's limitations and potentials.[16]

The social environment in any setting (education, rehabilitation, recreation, work) can have an impact on the acceptance and inclusion of people with disabilities. Creation of a positive social environment is a basic key to the successful integration of disabled people in community living, and the social atmosphere that recreation professionals create can influence the quality of social interaction between disabled and nondisabled people. Turnbull and Schulz have identified three factors which characterize a positive social atmosphere that can facilitate social integration in educational settings. These three factors are universal and are certainly applicable to recreation settings.

1. Open and Honest Communication

acknowledge strengths and weaknesses
acknowledge similarities and differences
explain inappropriate behavior
answer questions about disabilities
provide accurate information about disabilities, adaptive devices, etc.

2. Success

individualize instruction when possible
provide support and encouragement
recognize and acknowledge successes

3. Respect

tolerate differences
value the individuality of each human being
provide disabled people with status positions in programs
capitalize on the strengths and interests of all participants
provide opportunities for people to discover common interests and skills
facilitate "two-way" helping relationships between disabled and nondisabled people.[17]

The integration of disabled and nondisabled people into the mainstream of society is a means of achieving acceptance. Integration has been defined by Wolfensberger, who makes an important distinction between physical and social integration.

The author states:

> If integration is one of the major means for achieving and acknowledging social acceptance, as well as for accomplishing adaptive behavior change, then we must distinguish between and elaborate upon its dimensions and components. First of all, let us define integration as being the opposite of segregation; and the process of integration as consisting of those practices and measures which maximize a person's (potential) participation in the mainstream of his culture. . . . Ultimately, integration is only meaningful if it is social integration; i.e., if it involves social interaction and acceptance, and not merely physical presence. However, social integration can only be attained if certain preconditions exist, among these being physical integration, although physical integration by itself will not guarantee social integration.[18]

The process of integration that Wolfensberger describes involves the examination of physical and social environments. We have already identified the factors within the physical environment that can hinder the movement of disabled people into the mainstream of community life. Moreover, we have discussed, in general terms, the importance of a positive social environment in achieving social interaction. Let us now turn our attention to the specific factors in the social environment that can have a negative impact on the development of individuals with disabilities.

society's negative attitudes
social segregation
low social status and social roles
lack of appropriate rehabilitation
negative stereotypes found in media
limited social opportunities
overdependent parental influence
limited community opportunities
communication
discriminating policies and practices of organizations
low expectations placed on disabled people

At one time or another we have all felt lonely. We no doubt discovered that this feeling was one which we didn't want to feel very often. Loneliness is thought of as the "psychological state resulting from dissatisfaction with the number and quality of one's social and emotional relationships."[19] In a recent study which examined the relationship among loneliness, self-concept, and adjustment, the researchers found that "feeling lonely despite the potential availability of others may derive from a restricted and negative view of self."[20]

Successful and positive interaction between disabled and nondisabled people will have a direct influence on the self-concept of disabled people. Experiences that promote positive social interaction are very important, especially when the two groups are interacting with one another for the first time.

Promoting successful social interaction sometimes requires planned intervention on the part of the professional. When disabled people have equal roles in a reaction experience, both parties are able to show respect toward one another. For example, cooperative play experiences can often have a positive impact on an individual's self-concept.[21] Cooperative play experiences between disabled and nondisabled people result in higher self-esteem, personal acceptance, and more friendly interactions between the two groups.[22]

Ethnic and cultural factors.   Culture, ethnicity, and race provide a significant influence on how individuals perceive life, on the values they hold most highly, on their belief systems, their customs, and their behaviors. Every one of us is, in fact, bound by a set of culturally related values, beliefs, rules, and guidelines that are so much a part of us that they are nearly invisible to us.

How one copes in this context, with an illness or disability, is certain to be strongly influenced by these cultural parameters. Members of certain populations, for example, may rely on folk medicine for healing. For others, religion or being surrounded by certain objects with supposed supernatural power may be important.

Sometimes the differences in belief systems or behaviors between the consumer and the professional trigger difficulty. Unfortunately, most professionals are not racially or culturally literate. That is, when faced with unfamiliar and seemingly "nonsensical" consumer practices, professionals feel awkward or threatened. Similarly, members of racial or ethnic minorities may resist accepting helping services provided by members of the white race. Thus, we can see how differences in communication, both verbal and nonverbal, can create real barriers in therapeutic settings.

It would be dangerous to attempt to identify the predominant perspective of various ethnic and racial groups toward disability, rehabilitation, and coping. That could only result in stereotypes. Although a powerful influence, this perspective is only one of many factors affecting an individual's coping style. We must remind ourselves to identify our own cultural perspective, acknowledge those of others, and work toward achieving a multicultural perspective.

Role of the Family

The family, a small, interdependent social system that is undergoing change and redefinition, still remains a powerful social force. We have all experienced this social system and have felt its influence, for it has been instrumental in the development of our values, morals, and personalities. Many of us can look back upon this influence and remember positive, productive, and meaningful experiences. Others, unfortunately, will reflect upon their childhood with anxiety, fear, and anger.

The role of the healthy family implies understanding and acceptance of its members. The members of a family unit who support each other with love and caring may be able to cope with our rapidly changing society in a more productive manner. Leo Buscaglia offers some valuable insight regarding the meaning of the role of the family. The author states:

> Basically, then, the role of the stable family is to offer a safe training ground for the young child to learn to be human, to learn to love, to build his unique personality, develop his self-image and to relate with, and to, the changing greater society of which and to which he is born. To varying degrees, families succeed or fail in aiding the child toward the realization of these vital functions. Nevertheless, the child will grow into adulthood with or without these learnings and will have to deal with whatever the results. He may never be able to adjust to society or he may learn the necessary skills later, relearn them, or unlearn them, depending upon the pressures he is capable or willing to deal with in the processes involved in his self-actualization.[23]

The role of the families of disabled children carries with it the same responsibility and commitment charged to families of nondisabled children. There is, however, evidence suggesting that the problems faced by a family unit will be intensified when one of the members has a disability. The best way to understand the role of the family of the disabled person is in a social-psychological context. Viewing the whole environment and structure of the family unit allows us to evaluate the psychological state of a family as its members interact with one another, the community, and the larger society.

In the preceding section, the role of the family of the nondisabled person was highlighted by a quote from *The Disabled and their Parents: A Counseling Challenge*, by Leo Buscaglia. It seems appropriate, then, when discussing the role of the family of the disabled person to include a statement from the same book in which Buscaglia describes the responsibility faced by such a family. The author states:

> The family of the disabled can act in a most positive manner as a mediator between society in which the child will have to function and the more loving and accepting informed environment it can afford him. But to do this each family member must adapt to his own feelings about the disability and the child who is disabled. He must understand that only in this way can he help the child adapt to his feelings regarding his disability and finally, himself, as a total person.[24]

The process of adjustment to a disability is closely related to the attitudes and values of the disabled person, significant others, and society at large. The problems involved with the social-psychological adjustment to a disability are unique to each individual and family unit. In addition, there appear to exist several general characteristics of social-psychological response to disability that have implications to adjustment for the family unit. These general problems to adjustment are listed below to help the reader gain an understanding of the impact interpersonal relationships and societal pressures can have on an individual's ability to adjust to a disability.

> low social status
> physical and social insecurity
> parental attitudes and interaction
> family reactions and feelings
> lack of societal acceptance
> marital stress
> personal acceptance and adaptation
> limited knowledge of community resources
> self-concept
> socialization
> productivity and self-motivation

Sexuality and Disability

Social-sexual relationships are an integral part of every individual's growth and development. We live in a world where friendships, intimate relationships, marriages, and families allow us to express our emotions; sharing love and warmth becomes a fulfilling and gratifying experience. Even when social and emotional difficulties are present in our interpersonal relationships, we continue to strive for meaningful intimacy with these significant people in our lives. This need for love, belonging, and even self-esteem are basic human needs that we all strive to fulfill and satisfy.

The majority of human beings seek to satisfy their needs for affection and love without undue conflict or rejection from society. Myths regarding the nonsexuality of people with disabilities are evident in society's negative attitudes toward this minority group. Discrimination and ridicule regarding people with disabilities have placed a stigma upon this segment of the population.

The impact of society's negative attitudes on the social-sexual development of disabled people has been clearly documented. Charles Dunham explains this impact in a sensitive and realistic manner. The author states:

> Prejudicial thinking and active suppression have combined to deprive them of a successful sexual existence, one that meets their need not only for physical stimulation and satisfaction, but for a feeling of self-worth and acceptance, expressions of tenderness, and a sharing of both the joys and sorrows of life with a loved one. One of the greatest obstacles to achievement of these enriching relationships is the idea that the disabled are not sexual beings, that they are of neuter gender. Myths of nonsexuality surround spastic, blind, deaf, paraplegic and retarded individuals, just as they are imposed upon children and the elderly. Too often these myths have the effect of denying the disabled the

very foundations on which social-sexual life is built—early experience with the opposite sex, masturbation without guilt, basic information on the "facts of life," and the privacy that is necessary if romantic attachment is to develop.[25]

What is the basis for these negative attitudes? At least in the United States, Puritanism is a major reason for this negative response. This cultural influence accounts for the fact that society, historically and in some cases today, feels uncomfortable about the topic of sexuality in general and especially when disability enters into the conversation. Wolfensberger has identified five reasons which he feels undergird society's negative response toward disability and sexuality. These five reasons are summarized below:

1. Disabled people should not engage in sexual intercourse because this might result in impaired children.
2. Severely disabled people would be inadequate parents.
3. Individuals with disabilities are not fully human.
4. The general public appears to reject social-sexual relationships which they could not imagine for themselves.
5. Disabled individuals may not be able to meet certain marriage criteria.[26]

Obviously, these myths and stereotypes do not have any validity. Dispelling them, however, is not always an easy task. Accurate information and honest communication about sexuality and disability will certainly help. During the past decade the topic of human sexuality and disability has begun to appear in rehabilitation literature as well as in other helping professions. The following statistics from Isabel Robmault's *Sex, Society, and the Disabled* provide a glimmer of progress being made toward the tearing down of societal prejudice.

> About one of every ten persons of the general adult population has a disability which produces a physical handicap. Some of these handicaps had their onset at birth or in early childhood. Others have had an abrupt onset, while still others have had chronic progressive courses, starting before or after puberty and affecting the life-style of those so afflicted. However, in spite of common belief to the contrary, many disabled people report that their disabilities do not alter their sexuality or their libido. As so many careful observers are beginning to realize, sexuality remains as long as feelings (emotions) and imagination are intact.[27]

ENVIRONMENTAL FACTORS

The nature of disabling conditions and their impact on human development has been carefully studied. Specifically, various aspects of disability and certain characteristics of the environment have greatly influenced the social and psychological development of individuals with disabilities. Disabled individuals, like other people, cannot be fully understood if examined in a vacuum. The very nature of our existence implies constant and diverse interactions with other individuals, groups, cultures, and the environment as a whole. Understanding the impact a disability has on an individual can be fully realized only when individuals are perceived as developing human beings within the social and environmental context in which they interact.

The environment plays a particularly significant role in the development of all people. General environmental factors that can have major impact on the development of disabled people include the following:

1. *Architectural-Environmental:* location, physical context, size, access, appearance and internal design of residential, clinical, and community facilities.
2. *Transportation:* availability and usability of accessible public transportation.
3. *Support, Guidance, and Care:* degree of social and emotional deprivation in living, educational, working, or leisure environments.
4. *Mobility:* degree of independence to freely move through an environment.
5. *Adaptive Devices:* availability and usability of adaptive devices to increase independence.
6. *Information, Stimulation, and Motivation:* degree of meaningful and stimulating elements afforded by the environment.
7. *Security and Comfort:* degree of comfort and security afforded by the environment.
8. *Challenge and Risk:* degree of challenge and risk afforded by the environment.
9. *Teaching Elements:* degree and nature of teaching-learning elements incorporated into the environment.
10. *Age, Sex, and Physical Needs:* degree of appropriateness of the physical environment.
11. *Modification of the Environment:* degree of modification to the environment and the availability of stimulating opportunities of daily living.

Instead of focusing on the individual and the nature of his or her disability as the only influence of behavior, we should examine carefully the environment of the individual. The meaning of human behavior is more relevant when observed in a variety of settings. Because a disability impacts on the life of an individual in many ways, it can be compounded by the above environmental influences.

PSYCHOLOGICAL FACTORS

The psychological development of individuals with disabilities is influenced by many factors. The process of personal growth is gradual and needs to be nurtured in order to occur. Learning can be a natural state, and with careful attention and an openness to experiences, personal growth can take root in an individual. Our very being is the essence of this growth: How we appear to ourselves and to the external world is a result of our psychological maturation. The next section of this chapter discusses this concept in more detail.

Self-Concept: Factors Affecting a Positive Image

As a person goes through the process of adjusting to a disability or accepting personal limitations, his or her *self-concept* plays a key role. Many factors influence the development of a positive self-concept. Achieving personal competence and fulfillment is possible when people view themselves in a positive manner. When limitations are accepted as a natural part of human existence and inaccurate societal expectations are ignored, individuals are free to discover themselves and strive to reach and even go beyond their potential. We often lock our unique abilities away for fear of failing; society responds by saying, "I told you so!" A positive self-concept will enable us to reach for our dreams and aspire to be the people we were meant to be.

Our ability to learn social skills often relates to the way we perceive ourselves, that is, our self-concept. If we view ourselves in a negative fashion it will be difficult for us to make contact and establish meaningful interpersonal relationships with others.

Canfield and Wells comment on the meaning of self-concept and its impact on our development. The authors state:

> Your self-concept is composed of all the beliefs and attitudes you have about yourself. They actually determine who you are! They also determine what you think you are, what you do, and what you become! It's amazing to think that these internal beliefs and attitudes you hold about yourself are that powerful; but they are. In fact, in a very functional sense, they are your self.[28]

Another definition of self-concept expands on the different components of the self, which are worthy of mention. Singh and Wagner explain:

> Self-concept is a complicated term that includes many different ideas of self, two of which are self-esteem and self-actualization. Self-esteem is essential for any individual. He must feel he has worth. Self-esteem is derived from two main sources: the self and other persons. Esteem is earned as one achieves certain goals, operates by certain values, or measures up to certain standards. These goals, standards, and values may be internal, external, or both. They may be established, regulated, and applied by the judging self, by others, or by both.[29]

As you can see, self-concept is a complex psychological construct. Its characteristics have been summarized by Epstein, who observes:

1. It is a subsystem of internally consistent, hierarchically organized concepts contained within a broader conceptual system;
2. It contains different empirical selves, such as body self, a spiritual self, and a social self;

3. It is a dynamic organization that changes with experience;
4. It develops out of experience, particularly out of social interaction with significant others;
5. It is essential for the functioning of the individual that the organization of the self-concept be maintained;
6. There is a basic need for self-esteem, which relates to all aspects of the self-system;
7. The self-concept has at least two basic functions: (a) it organizes the data of experience, and (b) it facilitates attempts to fulfill needs.[30]

Love

Loving oneself is the most fundamental foundation for developing a positive self-concept. Love implies concern, caring compassion, and respect. People are not able consistently to extend these feelings or behaviors to other people if they don't hold these feelings for themselves. Leo Buscaglia offers a beautiful description of the impact love can have on individuals. The author states:

> If you know, accept, and appreciate yourself and your uniqueness, you will permit others to do so. If you value and appreciate the discovery of yourself, you will encourage others to engage in self-discovery. If you recognize your need to be free to discover who you are, you will allow others their freedom to do so, also. When you realize you are the best you, you will accept the fact that others are the best they. But it follows that it all starts with you. To the extent to which you know yourself, and we are all more alike than different, you can know others. When you love yourself, you will love others. And to the depth and extent to which you can love yourself, only to that depth and extent you will be able to love others.[31]

Love implies action, responsibility, and honesty with ourselves and others. Love is an experience. When touched by this experience we often feel a tug at our hearts or a connectedness with ourselves and others. As Buscaglia suggests, love begins with ourselves, and our active ability to share this experience with others depends on how well we know and love ourselves.

When the power of love is freely extended to us, or when we extend ourselves to others, we create a positive effect. These experiences over time can have an influence on our self-concept. A basic human need is to love and be loved. Love can open up possibilities for growth and change and help us to reach beyond our grasp, explore new experiences, and learn to function more effectively. Sidney Jourard describes one aspect of the loving experience:

> When I love—myself, family, friends—I see them in a special way. Not as the product of what they have been, or their heredity and schooling, though I notice that. I see them as the embodiment of incredible possibilities. I "see," imaginatively, what they might become if they choose. In fact, in loving them, I

may invite them to activate possibilities that they may not have envisioned. I lend them my creative imagination, as it were. If they are weak, I invite them to invent themselves as stronger and to take the steps necessary to actualize their latent strength. If they have been shy or self-concealing, I invite them to try on boldness and self-disclosure for size, to be more creative artist-of-them-selves. I too can be the artist-of-myself, if I love myself.[32]

Self-Disclosure

The concept of *self-disclosure* means "opening up to others."[33] Having someone to confide in or just talk to helps us deal with personal problems or life's stresses. It is apparent that self-disclosure not only is a necessary ingredient for establishing close relationships with others but it also helps us adjust to changes in our lives. Jourard, in his research, found that there is a positive relationship between self-concept and self-disclosure. The ability to be open with other people and reveal personal feelings and thoughts in a genuine manner is a characteristic of an effectively functioning personality.[34]

A healthy personality is characterized by a positive self-concept. One means of achieving a healthy personality, according to Jourard, is by allowing our real self to be visible to others. He writes:

> Self-disclosure is a symptom of personality health and a means of achieving healthy personality. When I say that self-disclosure is a symptom of personality health, I mean a person who displays many of the other characteristics that betoken healthy personality will also display the ability to make himself fully known to at least one other significant human being. When I say that self-disclosure is a means by which one achieves personality health, I mean it is not until I am my real self and I act my real self that my real self is in a position to grow. One's self grows from the consequence of being. People's selves stop growing when they repress them.[35]

Openness between disabled and nondisabled people, when both groups allow their real selves to be exposed, has the potential of enabling people to learn about their similarities and differences. This knowledge can perhaps lead to understanding and acceptance. The first step, however, is for all of us to take the risk of exposing our thoughts, feelings, and fears to one another. The ability to do this certainly must come from an attitude of trust and compassion. Being "real" is often a difficult concept to understand and apply. We live in a world where we have been conditioned to believe that we need to protect ourselves and our image. Self-disclosure is clearly a personal choice, a decision that each of us has to make on our own. Margery Williams, in her beautiful children's story *The Velveteen Rabbit*, has perhaps best described what it is like to be real. She writes:

> "What is real?" asked the Rabbit one day, when they were lying side by side near the nursery fender, before Nana came to tidy the room. "Does it mean having things that buzz inside you and a stick-out handle?"

"Real isn't how you are made," said the Skin Horse. "It's a thing that happens to you. When a child loves you for a long, long time, not just to play with, but really loves you, then you become Real."

"Does it hurt?" asked the Rabbit. "Sometimes," said the Skin Horse, for he was always truthful. "When you are Real you don't mind being hurt."

"Does it happen all at once," like being wound up," he asked, "or bit by bit?"

"It doesn't happen all at once," said the Skin Horse. "You become. It takes a long time. That's why it doesn't often happen to people who break easily, or have sharp edges, or who have to be carefully kept. Generally, by the time you are Real, most of your hair has been loved off, and your eyes drop out and you get loose in the joints and very shabby. But these things don't matter at all, because once you are Real you can't be ugly, except to people who don't understand."[36]

Locus of Control

Self-determination is a basic human right, but disabled persons are often stripped of this right by society. When disabled people are deprived of their right to make self-determined choices they are less able to learn from their experiences. Thus, when people lose a measure of control over their own lives, their self-concept is diminished.

The construct of *locus of control* was developed within social-learning theory, and it has been a major focus of study for the past two decades. Sawrey and Telford offer a simple definition of the term *locus of control*. The authors state:

> The external versus internal locus describes the degree to which a person believes that he possesses or lacks the power to control the events or circumstances of his life. More specifically, it refers to the extent to which the individual believes that the successes and failures in his life occur as the result of his own actions, on the one hand, or the outcomes of chance or luck, on the other.[37]

Research indicates that external control is related to low self-esteem, hopelessness, and depression. Many factors, as we have seen, can have an effect on disabled people. Most of these factors within the social and physical environment are external, which means they are outside of ourselves. When something is external, changing it is often beyond our control. We certainly have control over trying to change it, but we must ultimately realize that what is within our control are our attitudes and our ability to accept certain situations and change the manner in which we perceive them and control how the situation may influence our behavior.

It is easy to look at external variables to account for our difficult circumstances. It is also difficult to believe that we can have control and then take control over how we choose to respond to those difficult circumstances in our lives because of the nature of our conditioning. Many of us are not aware of the internal knowledge we have of ourselves and our experiences. The extent to which we can look inward and rely on our own knowledge depends a great deal upon our personal awareness and willingness to act and risk.

SUMMARY

Throughout this chapter we have explored the nature of disability by examining the social-cultural, environmental, and psychological factors that impact on the lifestyle of the person with a disability. By understanding these influences on human development, therapeutic recreation specialists can design services that espouse the ecological perspective of service delivery. Along with this understanding comes a respect for, and recognition of, the disabled individual as a whole human being.

The process of adjustment and coping with a disability was also discussed. The issues of self-concept and social support were included in this discussion to further illustrate that adjustment and coping are not thought of as a pragmatic approach to human existence, but rather, a process that demands personal strength and determination. The nature of disability is multifaceted and involves the dynamic interrelationship among the major factors presented in this chapter.

DISCUSSION QUESTIONS

6-1. What factors affect an individual's ability to cope with and adapt to his or her disability?

6-2. What is the potential impact of *labeling* on an individual?

6-3. What factors contribute to a positive social atmosphere?

6-4. What is the role of the family in assisting an individual to cope with a disability?

6-5. How is one's sexuality affected by disability?

6-6. How is one's self-concept developed? How does self-concept affect the coping process? How does disability affect self-concept?

6-7. What is meant by "locus of control"? This is an important concept in therapeutic recreation. We will come across it again and again. Be certain to understand its importance.

6-8. What role do you think a therapeutic recreator can play in assisting individuals to cope with their disabilities?

NOTES

1. Leo Buscaglia, *The Disabled and Their Parents: A Counseling Challenge* (Thorofare, N.J.: Charles B. Slack, Inc., 1975), p. 179.

2. Kathleen Collard, and others, *Closing the Gap: An Inservice Training Guide for Mainstreaming Recreation and Leisure Services* (San Jose, Calif.: San Jose State University, Department of Recreation and Leisure Studies, 1980), p. 85.

3. John Adams and Erich Lindemann, "Coping with Long-term Disability," in *Coping and Adaptation*, eds. George Coelho, David Hamburg, and John Adams (New York: Basic Books, 1974), pp. 127–138.

4. James Calhoun and Joan Ross Acocella, *Psychology of Adjustment and Human Relationships* (New York: Random House, 1978), p. 20.

5. James Sawrey and Charles Telford, *Adjustment and Personality* (Newton, Mass.: Allyn and Bacon, 1975), p. 73.

6. Sidney Cobb, "Social Support as a Moderator of Life Stress," *Psychosomatic Medicine*, 38, No. 5 (1976), 300–314.

7. Don Gibbons and Joseph Jones, *The Study of Deviance: Perspectives and Problems* (Englewood Cliffs, N.J.: Prentice-Hall, 1975), p. 3.

8. Constantina Safilios-Rothschild, *The Sociology and Social Psychology of Disability and Rehabilitation* (New York: Random House, 1970), pp. 114–115.

9. Mildred Blaxter, *The Meaning of Disability* (New York: Neale Watson Academic Publications, Inc., 1976), p. 13.

10. Kate Long, *Johnny's Such a Bright Boy, What a Shame He's Retarded* (Boston: Houghton Mifflin Co., 1978), p. ix.

11. Kenneth S. Thurman and Michael Lewis, "Children's Response to Differences: Some Possible Implications for Mainstreaming," *Exceptional Children*, 45, No. 6 (March 1979), 468–469.

12. John McDavid and Herbert Harari, *Social Psychology: Individuals, Groups, Societies* (New York: Harper & Row, 1968), p. 39.

13. Lee Snyder, Tony Apolloni, and Thomas Cooke, "Integrated Settings at the Early Childhood Level: The Role of Non-Retarded Peers," *Exceptional Children*, 43, No. 5 (February 1977), 262–266.

14. Candida Peterson, James Peterson, and Georgia Scriven, "Peer Imitation by Non-Handicapped and Handicapped Preschoolers," *Exceptional Children*, 43, No. 4 (January 1977), 223–224.

15. Michael Teague, "The Shangri-La Effect: Its Implications to Leisure Practitioners, "*Therapeutic Recreation Journal*, XII, No. 1 (1978), 23.

16. Buscaglia, *Disabled and Their Parents*, p. 177.

17. Ann P. Turnbull and Jane B. Schulz, *Mainstreaming Handicapped Students: A Guide for the Classroom Teacher* (Boston: Allyn & Bacon, 1979), pp. 345–354.

18. Wolf Wolfensberger, *The Principle of Normalization in Human Services* (Toronto, Canada: National Institute on Mental Retardation, 1972), pp. 47–48.

19. Ruth Ann Goswick and Warren H. Jones, "Loneliness, Self-Concept and Adjustment," *The Journal of Psychology*, 107 (March 1981), 237–240.

20. Ibid., pp. 237–238.

21. Roger Johnson, David Johnson, and John Rynders, "Effect of Cooperative, Competitive, and Individualistic Experiences in Self-Esteem of Handicapped and Non-Handicapped Students," *The Journal of Psychology*, 108 (1981), 31–34.

22. Linda Martino and David Johnson, "Cooperative and Individualistic Experiences Among Disabled and Normal Children," *The Journal of Social Psychology*, 107 (April 1979), 177–183.

23. Buscaglia, *Disabled and Their Parents*, pp. 74–75.

24. Ibid., p. 80.

25. Charles Dunham, "Social-Sexual Relationships," in *Disability and Rehabilitation Handbook*, ed. Robert M. Goldenson (New York: McGraw-Hill, 1978), pp. 28–29.

26. Wolfensberger, *Principle of Normalization*, p. 167.

27. Isabel Robmault, *Sex, Society, and the Disabled* (New York: Harper & Row, 1978), p. 166.

28. Jack Canfield and Harold C. Wells, *100 Ways to Enhance Self-Concept in the Classroom: A Handbook for Teachers and Parents* (Englewood Cliffs, N.J.: Prentice-Hall, 1976), p. 1.

29. Silas Singh and Tom Wagner, "Sex and Self: The Spinal Cord-Injured," *Rehabilitation Literature*, 36, No. 1 (1975), 2–10.

30. S. Epstein, "Self-concept Revisited: Or a Theory of a Theory," *American Psychologists*, 28 (1973), 404–416.

31. Leo Buscaglia, *Love* (New York: Fawcett/Crest, 1972), pp. 143–144.

32. Sidney M. Jourard, *The Transparent Self* (New York: Van Nostrand Reinhold Company, 1971), p. 55.

33. Arthur Nikelly, *Achieving Competence and Fulfillment* (Monterey, Calif.: Brooks/Cole Publishing, 1977), p. 40.

34. Sidney M. Jourard, *Self Disclosure: An Experimental Analysis of the Transparent Self* (New York: John Wiley & Sons, 1971), pp. 27–30.

35. Ibid., p. 32.

36. Margery Williams, *The Velveteen Rabbit* (Boston, Mass.: David R. Godine, Inc., 1983), pp. 4–6.

37. James Sawrey and Charles Telford, *Adjustment and Personality*, pp. 268–269.

TABLE 7-3 Effects of Hearing Loss

ASSOCIATED TERMS	EFFECTS OF LOSS ON UNDERSTANDING OF LANGUAGE AND SPEECH	PROGRAM IMPLICATIONS AND NEEDS
Slight to mild hearing impairment (Hard of hearing)	May have difficulty hearing faint or distant speech May experience difficulty with vocabulary and speech Understand conversations within 3 to 5 feet May exhibit speech defects and limited vocabulary	May benefit from hearing aid Proper lighting and close proximity to speaker will help Will benefit from hearing aid Attention to placement of person in relationship to speaker as well as proper lighting is necessary Fatigue and extraneous noise will affect person's ability to comprehend speech
Moderate hearing impairment (Hard of hearing)	Speech must be loud and distance small for person to comprehend conversation; will have difficulty unless conversation is directed at him or her Similar to above effects	Will need hearing aid Will need assistance to comprehend new vocabulary, concrete examples, and demonstration Close proximity to speaker and proper lighting are essential along with minimum background noise
Severe hearing impairment (Severely hard of hearing)	Understands only strongly amplified May hear voices about one foot away Speech is distorted; may be able to hear vowels, but not all consonants Speech and language defects present	Person will experience more difficulty in a group discussion Person will experience more difficulty in a group discussion Will need to be clued into topic; should face the speaker May benefit from interpreter for certain activities
Profound hearing impairment (Deaf)	Maximally amplified speech not understood May not hear loud sounds but is aware of vibrations Relies on vision rather than hearing as primary communication source	Person may need assistance of an interpreter, depending on the activity Demonstration and the use visual aids are essential New vocabulary must be taught

Chart adapted from H. David and S. R. Silverman (eds.), *Hearing and Deafness,* 3rd ed. (New York: Holt, Rinehart, and Winston, 1970); Illinois Commission on Children, *A Comprehensive Plan for Hearing-impaired Children.* (Springfield, Ill.: Office of the Superintendent of Public Instruction, 1968).

to moderate hearing losses. Thus, they will benefit from the same techniques outlined under speech reading although most will not learn to speech-read.

Manual communication. Sign language or finger spelling is one means through which some hearing-impaired persons communicate with others. *Manual communication* represents gestures, facial expressions, and body language in addition to sign language. An interpreter can be used during an activity to assist those hearing-impaired people who rely on sign language.

Speech reading. The process of visually identifying what a person says by watching not only the formation of the lips but also facial expressions and body movements is termed *speech reading* or *lip reading.* Because many sounds look identical on the lips, supplemental clues are important. Speech reading is a two-way process. The leader can do many things to make it easier for a hearing-impaired person to speech-read.

1. Speak clearly and at a moderately slow rate but do not exaggerate speech.
2. Face the hearing-impaired person directly and on the same level. Remember, speech reading is impossible beyond 8 to 10 feet.
3. See that light is not shining in the eyes of the person and that sufficient light is available.
4. Clue the person into a group discussion by telling the person what topic is being discussed.
5. Be expressive! Give the other person a key to how you are feeling by your face, eyes, and gestures.
6. If you eat, chew, or smoke while you talk, your speech will be more difficult to understand.
7. If a person does not reply or seems to be having trouble understanding, rephrase your words another way. You may have chosen words that are difficult to speech-read. Because context is important, avoid using single words.
8. Don't be afraid to write messages on paper.
9. Try to keep background noise to a minimum. If the activity will take place in a noisy environment, give key directions before in a quieter location.
10. Visual aids such as diagrams, written instructions, pictures, or media, in addition to verbal instructions, assist hearing-impaired individuals' comprehension of directions.
11. Because vocabulary comprehension is often limited, be sure essential words contained in directions and elsewhere are understood. Be sure the various steps of the game or activity and the sequence of these steps are understood before starting the game or activity. Enlist the assistance of parents, teachers, or other professionals to work with the participant on essential vocabulary words.
12. Because speech reading requires a great deal of concentration, alternate activities that require a great deal of communication with less-demanding activities.

Interpreters. Some individuals who are deaf may require the assistance of an interpreter to comprehend communication fully. Interpreters translate spoken words into sign language. Oral interpreters may be needed in a large-group setting to sit near deaf individuals who only use speech reading and not sign language. This type of interpreter translates verbal messages into words that are more easily distinguishable on the lips. Check with your branch of the local Department of Rehabilitation or Social Service for assistance in locating interpreters.

Telecommunications devices. These refer to various keyboard communication devices used by persons with hearing impairments to communicate visually over telephone lines. Teletypewriters (T.T.Y.) or computer-based systems are available. If such devices are not available at your agency, check with the local Social Services department or agencies that serve the deaf to see if they will give out needed information about recreation programs.

Hearing Aids

Hearing aids amplify sounds; yelling at a hearing-impaired person may hurt his or her ears. If a person's hearing aid is giving off a squeaking sound, inform the person so he or she can adjust the ear mold or the volume. The person may not be able to hear the squeaking noise. The volume-control switch on hearing aids can be turned down or off. On occasion, children with hearing impairments may intentionally tune you out. Check the volume switch. An extra battery on hand might also be wise. Hearing aids are delicate instruments; they should not be worn in water.

VISUAL IMPAIRMENTS

Visual impairments tend to be associated with many myths and stereotypes because of our tendency to personalize the disability and see only the most restrictive side. Clarification of terms is important to increase awareness of the range of visual impairments and to help dispel myths frequently associated with blindness. "It is necessary to know that the majority of visually impaired people are not totally blind, but are able to make use of residual vision or light perception. . . . "[15] Service providers will find it valuable to know how people with varying degrees of visual loss can function. Table 7–4 lists the different ranges of visual impairments.

Guidelines for Programming, Communication Skills, and Helping Techniques

The following guidelines will help therapeutic recreators to adapt a program, understand how to describe a situation or activity, and communicate more fully with a person who has a visual impairment.

TABLE 7-4 Ranges of Visual Impairments [Based on optimal visual correction]

ASSOCIATED TERMS OR DEGREES	FUNCTIONING LEVELS
I. BLINDNESS (LEGALLY BLIND)	
Total blindness: complete loss of vision and light perception (very small minority)	Will use braille and travel aids (cane, guide dog, and/or electronic aids)
No functional vision: Can see shadows or shapes but no details; sees shades of gray not black	Same as above
No peripheral vision: "tunnel vision;" sees the world as if looking through a hollow tube; must turn head in line with objects to see them	Can read regular print; independent mobility but may use optical aids for reading street signs; limited modification necessary for participation; has limited depth perception
II. PARTIAL SIGHT	
No central vision; cannot see what is "straight ahead" but can see peripherally as in macular degeneration	May use large-print books, magnification, aids, and/or braille; will have difficulty doing close-up work; may use cane
Blurred or cloudy vision; has difficulty focusing on objects, as with cataracts	May use braille, large-print books, and/or magnification aids; can usually travel independently without the use of aids
Limited ability to control the amount of light and accommodate to light changes; images appear "washed out"; few details can be detected	Wears dark glasses to protect eyes from bright light; may be a print reader with or without magnification aids
	(Any individual with a visual loss can benefit from talking books, tapes, records, etc.)

(Table adapted from: National Association for Visually Handicapped, Inc., "Classification of Impaired Vision," 1973; Anne Yeadon and Dava Grayson, *Living with Impaired Vision: An Introduction* (New York: American Foundation for the Blind, 1979).

1. Use descriptive language. People with limited vision must rely on others to describe the surrounding environment and fill in the gaps of what they don't see. Use descriptive language to describe events and the environment.
2. Orient the person with a visual impairment to new environments. Describe the size, boundaries, and any obstacles or potential hazards. If dominant cues are present, be sure to point them out.
3. When walking with a person who is blind, let the individual take your arm just above the elbow. Allow the person to walk a step behind you so that he or she can follow the motion of your body. Pause briefly before the steps and tell the person what is ahead and about the environment you pass.

4. Supplement predominantly visually oriented experiences with auditory and/or tactile cues.
5. When you enter a room where a blind person is, be sure to introduce yourself. Remember to let the person know when you leave the room so that he or she is not talking to an empty room.
6. Minimize background noise when instructing visually impaired individuals. Extraneous noise can be very distracting and create confusion for people who rely on auditory cues in their environment.
7. Loss of sight does not affect a person's mental ability. Talk directly to the person—not to others in their behalf.
8. Do not be afraid to use words like "see" and "look"; they are an integral part of our language, and people with visual impairments use them all the time.
9. When guide dogs are in their harness, they are working and must not be distracted. Be sure to ask permission before you pet or talk to a seeing-eye dog.
10. When walking with a person with a cane, walk on the opposite side of the cane.
11. When guiding people to their seats, simply place their hand on the back of the chair and let them seat themselves.

LEARNING DIFFERENCES

Mental Retardation

Most people mature in the same developmental sequence, but people differ in the rate at which they mature and how long they stay at each stage. People also differ in the amount of information they are able to process. Certain conditions affect the rate at which people process or learn the information they receive. One such condition is *mental retardation.*

Very simply defined, mental retardation is a condition in which general intellectual functioning is below that expected for chronological age. Basically, a person with this condition may take more time in going through any one developmental stage, depending on the degree and severity of mental retardation. A more complete definition includes the following three criteria:

1. IQ: significantly subaverage intelligence, below 70 IQ (100 IQ is average).
2. Adaptive behavior: deficits in adaptive behavior or the degree to which a person meets standards of personal and social responsibilities for one's age and culture.
3. Developmental period: The above criteria become evident before the age of 18.

Many common myths and stereotypes are associated with mental retardation. One of these myths is that all mentally retarded people are severely disabled. Table 7–5 lists the various levels of mental retardation, provides a brief description of various functioning abilities, and gives the approximate percentage of individuals who are "labeled" in each category.

TABLE 7-5 Levels of Mental Retardation

DEGREE/ASSOCIATED TERMS	FUNCTIONAL ABILITIES FOR ADULTS AGED 21 +	% OF ALL CON- SIDERED RETARDED
Mild/Educable	Capable of earning a living and participating fully in community life; may need advice about impor- tant decisions and eco- nomic matters	86–89
Moderate/Trainable	Capable of self-mainte- nance in unskilled jobs; simple, useful, repetitive work tasks under super- vision; can carry on sim- ple conversation and interact with others co- operatively	6–10
Severe/Custodial or Dependent	Can follow daily routines, perform repetitive tasks, and contribute partially to self-support under complete supervision	3.5
Profound/Life Support	Some motor and speech development; needs complete care and su- pervision for self-mainte- nance; interacts with others in group activities and simple games	1.5

Table adapted from H. J. Grossman, *Manual on Terminology and Classification in Mental Retardation,* 1977 revision (Washington, D.C.: American Association on Mental Deficiency, 1977).

Implications for Recreation

Persons with mental retardation respond well to the same effective in-structional strategies as one would use with any other individual. Beyond the general guidelines outlined at the end of this chapter, a few specific guide-lines should be noted:

1. Generally, people's ability to understand the speech of others will be more de-veloped than their own speaking vocabulary. Don't talk about the mentally re-tarded in front of them. As with speech impairments in general, a speech prob-lem may not be indicative of more limited intelligence. It could be related to a physiological problem.
2. Individuals with mental retardation are closest to the average population in the area of physical abilities. This is particularly true for people with mild mental

retardation. More time may be needed to learn new physical skills, but do not assume the person does not have the physical abilities.

3. The use of task analysis, carefully breaking down an activity into specific sequences, is a helpful technique. This enables the leader to teach small, sequential steps, provide sufficient repetition, and facilitate the successful learning of a new skill.

4. Social skill development is a key area to be stressed. Structured programs, positive role models, and firm rules for appropriate behavior are all techniques that will facilitate the interaction of nondisabled and mentally retarded people.

5. When giving directions use concrete language and examples; abstract language is more difficult to grasp.

Learning Disabilities

The term *learning disabilities* has many definitions; but basically it has come to mean the following:

1. That a person has an average or above average IQ. However, there is a discrepancy between a person's ability or potential and actual performance.

2. That the learning and/or behavior problems are not caused by other physical disabilities—visual, hearing, or motor impairments.

3. That emotional disturbance, cultural deprivation, or environmental disadvantages are *not* a major contributing factor.[16]

Essentially, people with learning disabilities do not fit our expectations about how people learn. They may be unable to learn to read, write, or spell as well as is expected for their age. In other words, some skills are good while others are low. Performance tends to vary from day to day.

TABLE 7–6 Learning Disabilities: Characteristics and Recreation Leadership Strategies

COMMON FUNCTIONING LEVELS	IMPLICATIONS FOR RECREATION
INTELLECTUAL FUNCTIONING	
May have long- or short-term memory problems	Build up skills gradually from simple to complex
Spoken language, thinking and written language may be quite delayed	Reduce the complexity of the directions; minimize unnecessary details
Reading, spelling, and arithmetic skills often are considerably below the norm	Explain the placement or use of each skill or strategy in the total game
	Some "overteaching" may be necessary, but be sure to make practice fun
	Use multisensory teaching strategies: Explain, demonstrate, and use visual aids to teach a new skill.

TABLE 7–6   [*Cont.*]

COMMON FUNCTIONING LEVELS	IMPLICATIONS FOR RECREATION

PERCEPTUAL SKILLS

May not know right from left, up from down, etc.	Demonstrate as well as explain directions
Awareness of positions, movements, and locations of body parts in relationship to each other may be poor	Speak slowly and use simple words during explanations
	Use color codes to help right-left discrimination
Figure-ground perception difficulties: May not be able to identify their teammates from the larger group	In team games, clearly differentiate team members by color
Auditory perception may be poor: can hear, but may misinterpret directions, especially multiple directions	Don't overemphasize competitive sports and activities; offer a wide range of experiences, including drama, art, music, etc.

BEHAVIOR-MOTOR FUNCTIONING

Excessive movement—can't sit still	Minimize "clutter" or distractions in the environment
Underactivity—avoids participation; is a loner	Establish clear rules and be consistent in their enforcement
Inflexible; becomes anxious when routines are changed	Avoid fatigue—don't overdo activities
Has difficulty changing to a new task.	Provide clearly defined spaces for participants to work
Spontaneous, impulsive behavior—doesn't think about consequences of behavior	Bring the activity to a complete end before beginning new one
	Allow time to wind down or for relaxation exercises after an active experience
Has coordination problems—jumping, skipping, throwing, catching, drawing, cutting with scissors	Lethargic participants may need extra warm-up activities to stimulate their interest and activity level
	Emphasize experiences that will help to develop social skills

Table adapted from Bryant Cratty, *Adapted Physical Education for Handicapped Children and Youth* (Denver: Love Publishing Company, 1980), pp. 174–182; H. Fried, "Plain Talk About Children with Learning Disabilities" (Washington, D.C.: Department of Health, Education, and Welfare, Publication No. (ADM) 79–825, June 1979); J. W. Lerner, *Children with Learning Disabilities* (Boston: Houghton Mifflin Co., 1976).

EMOTIONAL OR BEHAVIORAL DISABILITIES

Differences in emotional functioning are both expected and accepted in the daily lives of all individuals. Not everyone will respond the same to similar situations. Universally experienced "ups" and "downs" reflect people's efforts to satisfy the changing needs of each phase of life and to cope with the stresses associated with frustration and the demands of daily living. People adopt various coping strategies and personal styles of interacting with others.

Some people adopt emotional responses and behaviors that are perceived by others as inappropriate. Such behaviors and/or maladaptive coping strategies will tend to persist if people continue to receive reinforcement for their actions. This reinforcement can take the form of either positive or negative attention. For healthy change to occur, individuals must receive positive reinforcement for more productive behaviors. Remember that all people have the ability to learn new behaviors and coping skills.

Many definitions exist for emotional or behavioral disabilities. The essential features of most definitions include the following:

1. A consistent response to the environment in socially unacceptable and/or personally unsatisfying ways.[17]
2. Persistence of the maladaptive emotional or behavioral response.[18]
3. The severity or extent of the inappropriateness of the behavior according to the situation in which the behavior occurs.[19]

A therapeutic recreation specialist does not need to diagnose the type or cause of the emotional or behavioral difficulty in order to set up a program for individual needs and abilities. Rather, a specialist may focus on some of the following: the individual's style of interacting with others; the stresses experienced prior to the obvious behavior change; and the characteristics of the environment.

Individuals with emotional and behavioral disabilities are sometimes excluded from social situations and activities because other people hold vague fears about how the individual might possibly behave. Exclusion usually makes the problem worse because of the withdrawal of potentially positive reinforcement for appropriate actions. Table 7-7 contains information that

TABLE 7-7 Functional Abilities and Social Interaction

FUNCTIONAL LEVELS	ASSOCIATED BEHAVIORS	IMPLICATIONS FOR RECREATION
EMOTIONAL STRESS TOLERANCE LEVEL		
Refers to the person's ability to cope with stress or react to stress caused by changes in the environment or routines, with others, or interaction with authority figures.	The degree of severity of the behaviors will vary from one individual to another, from situation to situation.	Observe behaviors and try to determine antecedents of behavior. Consistency and acceptance. Let people know they are accepted but not a particular behavior. Suggestions below apply to *both* aggressive and passive behavior.

TABLE 7-7 [*Cont.*]

FUNCTIONAL LEVELS	ASSOCIATED BEHAVIORS	IMPLICATIONS FOR REC-REATION
EMOTIONAL STRESS TOLERANCE LEVEL		
1. Aggressive Behavior	Verbal and physical aggression, antisocial in nature	Establish rules for participant behavior with the group, discuss reasons for the rules and consequences of breaking them; keep limits clear, concise, and reasonable
	Impulsive, does not consider consequences of one's actions	Enforce rules consistently, reinforce positive behavior the first time if possible, then give warning
	Demanding, attention seeking	and enforce consequences established if behavior continues
		Provide cues to expected and appropriate behavior
	Defies authority	
	Destructive to self, others, or the environment	
	Quarrelsome, irresponsible	
2. Passive/Withdrawn Behavior	Lack of interest, daydreams	Don't stress competitive activities; emphasize cooperative experiences and allow time for solitary activities
	Low rate of social interaction	
	Timid, shy, sensitive, submissive	Balance program with active and passive activities
		Allow release of excess energy through physical activities; provide winddown and relaxation exercises
	Feelings of distress, expressed unhappiness	
	Fears of a general and specific nature	
	Lack of energy	
	Low self-esteem (tends to be true for most people with emotional and behavioral problems)	Provide opportunities for individual and group discussions which point out participants' strengths and common interests and feelings
		Provide structure and routine; a gradual reintro-

[*continued*]

TABLE 7-7 [*Cont.*]

FUNCTIONAL LEVELS	ASSOCIATED BEHAVIORS	IMPLICATIONS FOR REC-REATION
EMOTIONAL STRESS TOLERANCE LEVEL		duction of structure can be introduced as participants can tolerate it Build on strengths and interests Bring activities to a complete close before moving on to a new one
AWARENESS OF REALITY	Excessive expression of fantasy	Be honest about your tolerance of participants' behavior
	Confused, disoriented, forgetful	Do not encourage fantasy; ask questions that relate to here and now
	Short attention span, excessive daydreaming	Provide opportunities for success and positive attention from peers (important for most people)
	Lack of purposeful behavior	Be honest in communicating with participants; if you don't understand the person or the behavior, don't pretend to understand; discuss it with the person
	Behavior reflects poor judgment in terms of personal safety, anticipated reactions of others	Make sure you have people's attention before giving directions Give clear, specific directions Provide clear structure and limits to the activity
	Vague, evasive responses	
OTHER POINTS THAT APPLY:		Some individuals may be on medications; find out if medications are being taken and how they affect the person

TABLE 7-7   [*Cont.*]

FUNCTIONAL LEVELS	ASSOCIATED BEHAVIORS	IMPLICATIONS FOR REC-REATION
		Keep in mind that internal emotional conflicts are very draining of energy; balance active programs with more passive, relaxing ones

Table adapted from: C. S. Dunham, "Mental Illness, in *Disability and Rehabilitation Handbook*, ed. R. M. Godenson (New York: McGraw Hill, 1978); William I. Gardner, *Learning and Behavior Characteristics of Exceptional Children and Youth: A Humanistic Behavioral Approach* (Boston: Allyn & Bacon, 1977), pp. 383–409; L. A. Llorens, and E. Z. Rubin, *Developing Ego Functions in Disturbed Children: Occupational Therapy in Milieu* (Detroit: Wayne State University Press, 1967); A. Turnbull and J. Schulz, *Mainstreaming: A Guide for the Classroom Teacher* (Boston: Allyn & Bacon, 1979).

will enable service providers to recognize and build on functional abilities and stimulate successful social interaction. Keep in mind that many of the strategies mentioned can apply to any individual who is experiencing difficulty adjusting to the situation at hand.

GENERAL GUIDELINES FOR WORKING WITH PEOPLE

In addition to the guidelines and implications for therapeutic recreation discussed throughout this chapter, there are several other guidelines that can be applied to all participants. These guidelines offer general suggestions for working with people regardless of disability labels.

Personal Interaction Considerations

1. Consult with the experts—your participants—in order to determine potential programs or ideas on adaptations.
2. Never underestimate individuals' abilities. The principle of the "self-fulfilling prophecy" applies here. If you expect people to be successful, they are more likely to succeed. Conversely, if you expect them to fail, they have a greater tendency to fail.
3. Speak to participants, regardless of functioning levels, with respect and dignity.
4. Provide positive reinforcement to participants by describing in detail the nature of their successes. Provide support and encouragement during a failure situation. (Emphasize the importance of trying.)
5. Provide opportunities for participants to learn to value and accept individual differences.

Environmental Considerations

1. Minimize environmental barriers that limit functioning (for example, stairs, noise).
2. Crutches, wheelchairs, and prosthetic devices (such as artificial limbs) are necessary accessories. Do not take them away from participants unless they ask you to remove them. Nothing is more irritating than to have crutches taken away as soon as one sits down—leaving one stranded.
3. Find out as much as possible about special equipment, aids, or techniques that participants with physical disabilities use to assist them in daily living.
4. Provide adaptive equipment when necessary to include an individual in the experience. Staff can modify equipment or use commercially available adaptive equipment.

Instructional Considerations

1. Build on abilities to maximize independent functioning.
2. Focus program opportunities on building new interests, self-confidence, and social skills.
3. Provide opportunities for participants to perpetuate their natural curiosity and expand their creative abilities.
4. Use principles of activity and task analysis to facilitate the acquisition of leisure skills and a successful learning experience.
5. Recognize that individuals have different learning styles by incorporating multisensory aids when demonstrating new skills.
6. Provide challenges that match the ability level of participants, and minimize extrinsic reward to maximize the potential for "flow."[20]

SUMMARY

The underlying theme of this chapter is that our perceptions of people with disabilities tend to influence the type and quality of services provided. The behavioral-environmental approach suggested that service provision must recognize the interrelationship of people and their environments. The specific information presented on disabilities emphasized functioning levels and implications for recreation.

The importance of viewing disability as only one aspect of a person is poignantly illustrated by a story written by Laura, a sixth-grade youngster. In this vignette, Laura candidly acknowledges her strengths, limitations, and interests.

> I don't like cerebral palsy to be called a disease or an illness. I do not feel handicapped. Instead, I feel different, and everyone is unique. Here are some ways that I am different from other people:
>
> 1. I don't communicate verbally. I use my eyes, the expressions on my face, body language, and my Vista machine.
>
> 2. My arms and legs and the rest of my body don't always do what I want them to do. I am not sure if this is because my brain sent the right message

(same as anyone else's), but my body doesn't react to the message—or if my brain sends a different message and my body follows it.

Because of this, there are some things I don't do in the same way as other people do them. In order to get somewhere fast instead of running, I race along in my wheelchair. I need help to do some things that other people can do by themselves (eat, go to the bathroom, for example).

There are some things that I don't do at all that other people do (chew gum, eat jawbreakers).

In most ways I am the same as anyone else. I have favorite interests and hobbies—drawing, watching TV, reading, eating, playing games, visiting with friends, laughing, and joking. There are also things I can do that I don't like to do (eat liver for dinner).

DISCUSSION QUESTIONS

7–1. What are some of the criticisms of the traditional categorial approach to disabilities? Why is it important for therapeutic recreators to examine alternatives to this approach?

7–2. How would the "functional" and "behavioral" approaches to disability be helpful to therapeutic recreators as they plan for intervention with individuals and their environments?

7–3. Why is it important for all leisure-service personnel to acquire basic information regarding disabilities?

7–4. What are five general guidelines for working with people regardless of disability labels? How would you apply these guidelines in a recreation program?

7–5. Read again the vignette written by Laura at the end of this chapter. Discuss what you think Laura's philosophy of disability might be. Why is it important to understand an individual's strengths, limitations, and interests? Would there be any implications for recreation programming based on this information? How could the functional and behavioral approach to disability be helpful in working with Laura?

NOTES

[1]Jim Hammitt, "A Gift of Love," *Mainstream* (December 1980).

[2]Burton Blatt, "Mainstreaming: Does it Matter?" in *Implementing Learning in the Least Restrictive Environment: Handicapped Children in the Mainstream*, eds. John W. Schifani, Robert M. Anderson, and Sara J. Odle (Baltimore, Md.: University Park Press, 1980), p. 496.

[3]Robert M. Smith and John T. Neisworth, *The Exceptional Child: A Functional Approach* (New York: McGraw-Hill, 1975), p. 8.

[4]Ibid., pp. 8–9.

[5]William I. Gardner, *Learning and Behavior Characteristics of Exceptional Children and Youth: A Humanistic Behavioral Approach* (Boston: Allyn & Bacon, 1977), p. 52.

[6]Smith and Neisworth, *Exceptional Child*, p. 169.

[7]Gardner, *Learning and Behavior*, p. 193.

[8]Thomas A. Stein and H. Douglas Sessoms, *Recreation and Special Populations*, 2nd ed. (Boston: Holbrook Press, 1973), p. 16.

[9]Frank Bowe, *Handicapping America* (New York: Harper & Row, 1978).

[10]Gardner, *Learning and Behavior,* p. 37.

[11]M. P. Scott, "Epilepsy: An Update on Treating Brain Disorders That Can Afflict Anyone, Anytime," in *Exceptional Children: A Reference Book,* ed. Herbert Goldstein (Guilford, Conn.: Special Learning Corp., 1978).

[12]Bryant Cratty, *Adapted Physical Education for Handicapped Children and Youth.* (Denver: Love Publishing Company, 1980), p. 340.

[13]"The Greatest Tragedy" (National Epilepsy League: Chicago, Ill., n.d.)

[14]Max Ellenberg, "Diabetes Mellitus," in *Disability: A Rehabilitation Handbook,* eds. Robert M. Godenson, Jerome R. Dunham, and Charles S. Dunham (New York: McGraw-Hill, 1978), p. 354.

[15]Anne Yeadon and Dava Grayson, *Living with Impaired Vision: An Introduction* (New York: American Foundation for the Blind, 1979).

[16]Maynard C. Reynolds and Jack W. Birch, *Teaching Exceptional Children in All America's Schools* (Reston, Va.: Council for Exceptional Children, 1977), pp. 348–351.

[17]James M. Kauffman, *Characteristics of Children's Behavior Disorders* (Columbus, Ohio: Chas. E. Merrill, 1977), p. 23.

[18]Eli Bower, *Early Identification of Emotionally Handicapped Children in School,* 2nd ed. (Springfield, Ill.: Chas. C Thomas, 1969), p. 25.

[19]Ibid.

[20]Gary Ellis, Peter Witt, and Tersita Aguilar, "Facilitating Flow Through Therapeutic Recreation Service," *Therapeutic Recreation Journal,* 17, No. 2 (1983), 6–15.

8

THE EVOLUTION OF SERVICES TO PERSONS WITH DISABILITIES
Maintenance, Treatment, Education, and Integration

"I find this field so confusing," stated the frustrated student to his instructor and some peers. "The terms used to refer to the field even vary from therapeutic recreation to recreation therapy to leisure services for ill and disabled persons. Why is it?"

"Yeah," chimed in another student. "I guess it's because the field is so new, but I can't figure out how programs provided in clinical settings relate to community programs. And why are some programs very specialized and others integrated to include persons with and without disabilities. Can you explain?"

"I understand exactly how you feel," replied the teacher. "I have often been frustrated myself. I found that it helped me to understand how leisure services have been provided since early times and to look at therapeutic recreation services in context of what has been taking place in society at the same time. You may also be surprised to find out that leisure and recreation are as old as humankind itself and have been an integral part of life. It's not as new as you may have believed."

INTRODUCTION

Any discussion of the development of therapeutic recreation services is bound to be complex, for an analysis must include a recognition of the meanings of leisure, the societal response to disabled persons, and the development of intervention all within cultural and social contexts. Leisure services are a reflection of society itself, and they are influenced by forces present within a given culture within any time frame. Thus, a study of service delivery provides insight into the social, economic status, and political mood of society.

While it is not possible to present any more than a superficial overview of the evolution of therapeutic recreation services, major trends will be highlighted.

AN HISTORICAL PERSPECTIVE

Various forms of recreation have been documented throughout recorded history. From artifacts, such as remains of instruments, pieces of pottery, and paintings on walls representing every facet of life, it is apparent that music, visual arts, dramatic rituals, spas, games, and many other types of recreation were woven into the earliest societies. Several authors[1] suggest that there is evidence of integral weaving of recreation, health, and religion throughout history. The first section of this chapter will examine this relationship and allied issues from earliest times through the present age.

The Folk Era: Survival of the Fittest

Anthropologists tell us that disability and disease have existed since the first beginnings of humanity and were thought of as agents of a hostile world. In preliterate society, hunting and gathering were the major forms of survival. Clans traveled together to seek food and shelter. The 1982 film *Quest for Fire* suggested that the lives of the earliest people were preoccupied with maintaining fire, carrying it with them as they moved, and stealing it from others if some mishap squelched their own source of heat and light. In this rugged existence, each person was required to assume a role in sustaining and protecting the clan from harm. Within the simple organization of labor, those unable to contribute to survival were of little use to the tribe and were often left behind for the natural elements to take their toll.

Leisure and recreation were part of daily life, woven into rituals of dance and music, appeasing the good supernatural spirits and driving away those deemed evil. It was also through play that survival skills and cultural values were taught. The boy returning from his first successful hunt was promoted to adulthood through a celebration of his feat that was marked by dance, rhythmic music, and painted masks.[2]

In these primitive societies, rehabilitation had its beginnings. Natural mineral or hot water springs relieved the aching muscles of the workers. Heat, herbs, mud, and other naturally acquired materials were used for healing and soothing sores.

Agrarian Society

As tribes developed agricultural skills and began remaining in one place for longer periods of time, less effort was required for basic survival. The new freedom from constant survival efforts was evidenced in changing cultural patterns. New forms of art emerged, from decorated clay vessels to the decoration of clothes. New games were developed. Even new forms of intimacy could now be enjoyed.

Within ancient civilizations, the first writings reflect the beginnings of a literate society. Chinese society was highly developed, as demonstrated by beautifully crafted and decorated porcelain (whereas the remainder of the world ate from mud plates).

Recorded as early as 3000 B.C., the Chinese practiced a series of light exercises called Cong Fu to promote health and longevity.[3] Ancient Hindus laid out rules for medical and health professions. Today, we practice one of their contributions, yoga.[4]

In the advanced society of Egypt, we find evidence of the therapeutic activities, such as walks and gymnastics, integrated with magic of the priest–physician, a manifestation of the bonding of religion and well-being. The beautiful Egyptian temples, dedicated to mental health, were places to enjoy lotus gardens and songs.[5] The therapeutic potential of the environment was, thus, identified early in the development of human healing.

The Hammurabi code of "An eye for an eye; a tooth for a tooth" was accepted not only in Babylonia but in many ancient civilizations. Thus, compensation for injury and the beginning of penology were codified.

The Jewish concept of one God began to curb superstitions and belief in magic so evident throughout earlier history. Perhaps the perception that holiness and health were inextricable resulted in the notion that disease was punishment for sin. This belief still has manifestations in today's negative attitudes toward disabled persons, as discussed in earlier chapters.

Body and Mind Integrated

A leap of several centuries to the erá of Greek and Roman civilizations offers us insight into the development of rehabilitation, an understanding of leisure, and the relationship of both to disabled persons. The Greeks strived to attain perfection of body and mind and sought to understand humans through reason, as opposed to religion.

Excellence of body, mind, and spirit.   The emphasis on human perfection and the relationship of body and mind played an important role in the evolution of rehabilitation. Temples, similar to our contemporary health spas, catered to a balanced state of mental, physical, and spiritual well-being. An ancient "multiservice center," a temple called Epidaurus, provided a place of worship, lodging, hospital quarters, gymnasium, library, theater, and stadium facilities.[6]

Music, seen as having curative powers, was used in rituals. Apollo was god of music, poetry, and medicine, reflecting the linkage of recreation to health. The care of the body was essential because it was the temporal abode of the soul. Recreation, in its many forms, was used then to promote both a healthy body and a healthy soul.

Gymnastics were developed by Herodicus in 480 B.C. to remediate physical discomfort. His student, Hippocrates, the "Father of Medicine," was also credited with writing exercise books and treating each person based upon observation.[7] These remedial measures were used to relieve illness believed to be caused by natural circumstances. Hippocrates also made a major contribution to the development of rehabilitation by stressing the "case study" approach or the *individual* treatment rather than the mass care of patients.

The importance of recreation and leisure was apparent in classical Greece. Plato asserted the value of play and ritual in the 8th book of *Laws* in the fourth century B.C. Leisure was an integral part of life to the free citizens of Greece. Aristotle roughly defined leisure as "freedom from the necessity of labor" (*Politics,* Book 2). Certain leisure activities were considered so beneficial that towns were carefully planned to include provisions for important cultural and physical events. Sports, education, and the arts stressed the value of a sound body and mind. Unfortunately, leisure and culture were available to only a small segment of the society, namely free men. Denied equal access were women, slaves, the poor, and most likely, the disabled, with their imperfect bodies or minds. In Plato's *Republic,* one finds instructions on how to deal with "deformed" babies: They were to be left on a mountaintop as sacrifices. Thus, while leisure was highly valued and well developed in the most classical sense, those who were not valued in society had no access to it.

In Rome, leisure opportunities *were* available to the masses, particularly in the form of sometimes brutal spectator events and through community baths. These baths signaled a further development in rehabilitation, for they were used for exercises, hydrotherapy, and social interchange. According to one authority, an important contribution of the Roman Empire was the development of the hospital system.[8]

Effects of Christianity

With the decline of the Roman Empire, the single most important force affecting Western civilization was Christianity. It was through the authority and governance of the Christian Church that the scientific developments of prior eras were subjugated to an emphasis on faith. Temporal and secular expressions were abandoned and replaced by sacred, spiritual pursuits.

In leisure, this led to an appreciation of contemplation and prayer, and a condemnation of previous ritualistic activities, such as celebrations, dance and music, games, and so forth. Dogmatic religion preached by the Church proved triumphant.

Although disease was considered a result of natural causes in Greek and Roman eras, in Medieval Europe disease was once again viewed as having supernatural origins, thus setting back medical progress. Feudal lords were entertained by jesters who were often disabled persons. The greater the deformity, the greater the laughter they provoked from audiences. For perhaps the first time, disabled persons were "valued" economically, sought by the

wealthy for entertainment. Under these distasteful circumstances, these individuals were earning a living.

The Church assumed responsibility for providing custodial care for ill
and disabled persons within the walls of its monasteries. The Church also
built hospitals, but most medical care declined in favor of an emphasis on
spiritual well-being. Although little information is available on the life led by
individuals in the Church's care, it can be speculated that physical care may
have been accompanied by diversionary recreation. Actual treatment of the
disabled or educational opportunities for them probably did not become
available until the eighteenth century.

Later Developments

The eighteenth and nineteenth centuries saw a dramatic shift away
from the dogmatism of the Christian Church. Culture in its many forms was
encouraged to flourish.

Discoveries included voyages to the New World, a broader distribution
of knowledge via the printed word, and growth in scientific medicine. Human understanding and respect for personal freedom began to take root. Hu-
manitarianism was a predominant perspective, reflected in the many social
developments.

Colonial America: stress on individualism.   The evolution of the care
and treatment of disabled persons in the American colonies is noteworthy.
For the most part, disabled persons were the responsibility of their families.
Few provisions for assisting these individuals or their families were available
through the colonial government. The colonies adopted in principle the British poor law system, which localized public relief.

Hard work and physical stamina were human qualities thought to be
significant in attaining material success and spiritual worthiness, and they
were signs of societal progress. Those unable to work were merely tolerated.

Families, the basic foundation of colonial life, were responsible for their
members. Those individuals unable to perform required work functions were
dependent upon family members for their well-being. Colonial governments
attempted to curb the number of "dependents" coming to the New World.
When there were indications that Britain was sending over disabled individuals, the colonial administration would ask the mother country for a subsidy.
Those individuals without families who could care for them were "farmed
out" to other families by the colonial government. One Hadley, Massachusetts, resident was said to have boarded with 32 different families over a period of 65 weeks, certainly a disruptive life.[9]

Upon recovery from illnesses, those who were farmed out were expected to repay their host families during a period of indentured servitude.[10]
And although the governing authorities would assume some social responsibility for assisting dependent persons when necessary, an individual with
even modest means could be expected to relinquish all holdings to the local

community in return for public aid. It is, of course, important to remember that charities and endowed religious organizations did not exist in the early days of the colonies. The practices, then, reflected social conditions of the time.

As the population increased, with a majority of persons attracted to eastern, seaport towns in the eighteenth century, the need for alternate forms of care for poor and disabled persons emerged. Public almshouses developed to shelter dependents when the normal channels of family care were unavailable. These typically provided a minimal level of food and shelter to a mixed grouping of able-bodied poor, ill, and disabled persons. An almshouse was in existence in Boston as early as 1662.[11]

The reputation of almshouses today probably is not far removed from the reality of the situation. Myths and superstitions about disabled persons, the strong work ethic that rejected the poverty of well persons, the lack of a strong social consciousness in the midst of a country striving for basic survival—all contributed to the fear and notoriety surrounding the almshouses. The physical environs of these places were said to have been dungeonlike; the emotional environment was not any more humane. Records show that these places provided bizarre entertainment for the community. Cruel treatment, including the use of chains for restraints, led to the eventual outcry that demanded that changes be made in the almshouses in this country and in Europe.

One significant manifestation of a belief in the supernatural was the infamous witch trials, which sought to purge a community of "evil spirits." Often the victims of the scourge were women who exhibited behavior not thought to be appropriate. Today, some of that behavior might be considered symptomatic of mental illness. Other behavior is thought to resemble that of psychic healers today.

The first medical institution documented in America was the Pennsylvania Hospital, located in Philadelphia and established in 1751.[12] The services provided included those for mentally ill persons, who were previously denied treatment. Benjamin Franklin was one of the supporters of the hospital. However, there is evidence that the "treatment" afforded the mentally ill included brutality and rejection. Apparently superstition surrounding disease and disability continued to form the basis for treatment in both Europe and the United States.

There is evidence that the first medical speciality, orthopedics, developed in Switzerland in the 1700s,[13] and the first American hospital devoted exclusively to the care of the mentally ill was established in Williamsburg, Virginia, in 1773, in order to make provisions for the "Support and Maintenance of Idiots, Lunatics and other persons of Unsound Minds." The push for more institutional care for the mentally ill resulted from humanitarian efforts, scientific discovery, and the public fear of mysterious diseases.

Historically, colonies gave special consideration to war veterans and sea-

ual system of sign language, was in philosophical conflict with later schools that used the oral method of communication. Alexander Graham Bell became a leading spokesman for oral communication, experimenting with audio amplification systems.

Mental retardation emerged as a recognizable public concern in the 1800s. Perhaps the complexity of industrial and urban life, combined with greater social expectations, made those with retardation more conspicuous than was true in rural societies. The first private school to educate severely retarded individuals in America opened in Massachusetts in 1848. Its purpose was to promote the eventual participation of the students in their own communities. However, when efforts to move students back into their communities failed, the students who remained became permanent residents and the treatment changed from educational to custodial. Ironically, the humanitarian efforts to meet the needs of individuals through quality care unwittingly led to the creation of huge institutions, many of which still exist today.

Social Reform and the Roots of Organized Recreation Service

The formulation of social policy.   The demands of industrialism slowly eroded the quality of life in urban settings. Poverty was common, as were long days of hard, grueling work. Cities were beset with labor unrest, congestion, and filth. It was conditions such as these that spawned the progressive reform movement in the late nineteenth and early twentieth centuries. The thinking behind this movement stressed the importance of both the physical and social environment of people. Helen Keller, one of the spokespersons of the movement, forcefully propounded the need to alleviate poverty and labor exploitation and urged preventative measures and treatment as ways to deal with blindness.

The recreation and leisure-services movement emerged from the same humanitarian roots as did the efforts of social-reform pioneers. The basis for the efforts of recreation pioneers was a concern for the quality of life. They advocated improved living and working conditions to enhance physical, mental, and social well-being.

Settlement houses, such as the well-known Hull House in Chicago, established by Jane Addams in 1889, were a reflection of a heightened social consciousness and social responsibility on the part of upper-class and educated members of society. Programs encompassed social, educational, and recreational services for immigrant workers, unwed mothers, the hungry, sick, and aged. Settlement workers, pushing for environmental reform, organized labor unions for women garment workers and helped establish day nurseries for children of working families.

Joseph Lee, called the "Father of the American Playground Movement," established an experimental playground in response to the jailing of youngsters for playing in the streets.

But it was not until the presidency of Theodore Roosevelt, in the early years of the twentieth century, that the federal government responded significantly to correcting the nation's social ills. Among the social reform measures was the enactment of legislation designed to provide vocational rehabilitation for World War I veterans, and later, for civilians.

Advancements in rehabilitation.   In the scientific community, new advances were being made. In 1895, Wilhelm Roentgen discovered X rays. The French neurologist J. M. Charcot successfully identified the causes of cerebral hemorrhage. In psychiatry, Emil Kraepelin devised the first classification of mental illness, and Sigmund Freud introduced the psychotherapeutic approach to the treatment of mental disorders.

Treating the whole person through rehabilitation received serious attention. In 1906, Conrad Biesalski conducted a census of disabled children in Berlin. He was credited with the development of the first comprehensive rehabilitation center in the world, Oscar-Helene Heim.[21] The Cleveland Rehabilitation Center deserved credit for being the first to open its doors in the U.S. in 1889.

The first organization to study the overall problems of disabled individuals, the Bureau of the Handicapped of the New York City Charity Organization Society, was founded in 1908; and the first of today's voluntary organizations to be established was the National Society for Crippled Children and Adults.

In the 1920s and 1930s, many public schools began to offer specialized classes. And in institutional schools, a stronger emphasis on the education of disabled children was evident.

The Beginnings of Contemporary Recreation and Leisure Services for Persons with Disabilities

War again played an important role in advancing opportunities to disabled persons. As part of its charter, the American Red Cross developed a Division of Recreation in Hospitals to provide entertainment and basic recreation programs within military hospitals for those wounded in war. During the 1920s and 1930s, the number of medical organizations providing recreation programs increased, primarily in hospital settings. The value and use of recreation therapy was documented as early as 1937 at the Menninger Clinic, a famous center serving individuals with mental illness. One of the earliest documented research studies on the benefits of recreation appeared in 1932. Researchers reported that recreation was useful in developing social skills at the Lincoln State School and Colony in Illinois.[22]

In 1932, the Bill of Rights for the Handicapped, adopted by the White

lished in the early 1960s and revised in the late 1970s, attempted to standardize accessibility design.[31] Public Law 90–480, the Architectural and Transportation Barriers Act of 1968, established mandatory facility standards, using ANSI A117.1 as the basis for regulations. This act states that, "Any building constructed in whole or in part with Federal funds must be accessible to and usable by the physically handicapped."[32] The Architectural and Transportation Barriers Compliance Board, created by the Rehabilitation Act of 1973, was designed to enforce compliance with P.L. 90–480. Whereas public buildings and facilities are covered by law, private settings are not currently mandated by the federal government to meet accessibility standards. Thus, restricted mobility of some persons continues to exist in many community leisure settings, such as restaurants, theaters, cultural centers, museums and galleries, sport arenas, and health clubs.

What are the implications of a barrier-free environment (that is, an environment which allows for maximum independent mobility of all persons) for nondisabled persons? Generally, the architectural accommodations that were originally designed to increase mobility-independence for disabled persons, indeed, increased mobility-convenience for able-bodied persons. For example, for high-use mobility and recreation devices, such as bicycles, skateboards, baby carriages, and grocery pushcarts, convenience is increased with the use of ramps, curb cuts, and elevators. Other devices, such as door handles, as opposed to round door knobs, make it easier for individuals with arms full of books or groceries and individuals with limited hand movement to open doors. Accommodations for persons with disabilities are, in fact, conveniences and safety features for everyone. (Refer to Table 8–1.)

Leisure-service program accessibility.   Although facility accessibility was mandated in the 1960s, a need was demonstrated for legislation protecting disabled persons from other types of discrimination, particularly when it came to services. Disabled protestors staged a sit-in for 24 days at the Department of Health, Education and Welfare buildings in both Washington, D.C., and San Francisco to demand the signing and implementation of the Rehabilitation Act of 1973. This action resulted in a new public awareness of these individuals and the eventual signing of significant clauses of the act. Section 504, approved by the Carter administration in the summer of 1977, states: "No otherwise qualified individual in the United States shall solely by reason of his handicap, be excluded from participation in, be denied the benefits of, or be subjected to discrimination under any program or activity receiving Federal financial assistance."[33] This section is particularly important because it is the first major federal law that specifically protects the civil rights of disabled persons.

Education legislation.   Public Law 94–142, signed in 1975, mandated that mainstreaming be started in public schools by the 1977–1978 school year.

TABLE 8-1   Personal Implications of Architectural Barriers for Independence

---

Consider:
It is necessary for you to use a wheelchair to be mobile.

You find yourself at the bottom of a flight of steps and the class you are taking is on the second floor. No elevator. . . .

OR

The restaurant that you and your friends are going to for a social evening has a door too narrow for your wheelchair to roll through. . . .

OR

The only spot in the movie theater where you can sit in your chair is at the rear of the building. . . .

OR

The counter over which you need to transact business is above your head. . . .

Do these situations mean:

1. that you are mobility-impaired?

OR

2. that the environment is impairing your ability to be independent?

What are your alternatives at the moment you encounter these barriers?

1. Go home?
2. Try another class, restaurant, theater, business?
3. Have a friend or friends—or strangers—lift and carry you?
4. Suggest that the class be changed; the theater and restaurant and business adapt the environment?
5. Sue?
6. Other?

This law was designed to ensure that all handicapped children are provided a free and appropriate public education; and related services are to be provided to each child in the "least restrictive setting."

The Individual Education Plan, or IEP, which is a requirement of P.L. 94-142, is used to ensure that the needs and abilities of each child are attended to and recognized. This plan consists of a yearly child assessment, the identification of individual goals, behavioral objectives, facilitation and implementation processes, and evaluation criteria.

The law has important implications for the therapeutic recreation profession: Recreation is specified as a "related service."

These legislative actions represent a successful effort on the part of disabled consumers and parents of children and young people with disabilities. Legislation continues to be enacted at the state and national levels to ensure the rights of all persons with disabilities. Laws seem to have an attitudinal impact on society, as reported by various studies. In one study completed in 1978, a panel of recreation administrators in California was asked to respond to 188 guidelines on mainstreaming. Those guidelines identified by the administrators as being "essential" in the mainstreaming process focused on the elimination of architectural barriers, which is mandated by law. In the same study, a panel of school administrators rated as essential those guidelines that focused on the elimination of discriminating policies, elimination of labels, elimination of architectural barriers, and on the need to make a commitment to mainstreaming. Each of these principles reflected the mainstreaming efforts in education (through P.L. 94–142) at the time of the study.[34] Federal and state mandates play an important role in shaping societal attitudes and policies and in forming the basis of service delivery. A review of the most important laws is included in Table 8–2.

Today, consumers and their advocates continue to work to increase legislation that will help to improve the quality of life of persons with disabilities.[35]

TABLE 8–2   Legislating Rights for Persons with Disabilities

YEAR	LAW	IMPACT
1917	Smith-Hughes Law	Established Federal Board for Vocational Education
1918	P.L. 65–178	Provided physical and vocational rehabilitation for W.W.I. vets
1920	P.L. 66–236	Extended vocational rehabilitation benefits to physically disabled civilians
1943	P.L. 78–113 (Barden-LaFollette Vocational Rehabitation Amendments)	Amended 1920 act; broadened benefits to include physical, mental restoration; blind persons included in rehab; vocational training and placement included for mentally ill
1946	National Mental Health Act	Provided financial assistance
1950	39 states and Hawaii have legislation related to the education of physically handicapped children	
1954	Vocational Rehabilitation Amendments	Expanded 1943 provisions to include research and demonstration projects, training

(continued)

TABLE 8-2 [*Cont.*]

YEAR	LAW	IMPACT
1963	Rehabilitation Act Amendments	Added recreation for ill and handicapped persons to areas eligible for training program assistance
	P.L. 88–164 Mental Retardation Facilities	Legislated construction of facilities to serve persons with mental retardation
1965	Amendments to Mental Retardation law	Increased services for severely disabled; construction of sheltered workshops, rehabilitation centers, residential accommodations for mentally retarded persons
1967	P.L. 90–170	Established the Bureau of Education for the Handicapped (BEH)
1968	P.L. 90–480	Provided for the elimination of architectural barriers to physically handicapped persons; established mandatory facility standards
1973	P.L. 93–112 Rehabilitation Act of 1973	Comprehensive rehabilitation law; Section 504 prohibits discrimination in programs receiving federal funds; individual rehabilitation programs; established Architectural and Transportation Barriers Compliance Board
1974	P.L. 93–380 Education Amendments	Granted handicapped children additional rights with regard to education
1975	P.L. 94–142 Education for All Handicapped Children Act	Granted all handicapped children the right to a free and appropriate education in the least restrictive setting
	Developmental Disabilities Act	Persons with developmental disabilities have right to services in the least restrictive environments
1976	All states have laws subsidizing public school programs for exceptional children	
1978	P.O. 95–602 Rehabilitation Act of 1978	Authorized funds for integrating handicapped persons into existing programs (including recreation) and provided rehabilitation services for severely handicapped persons

Litigation: Rights of Disabled Individuals to Treatment and Education

Although some success in attaining equal access to services used by the disabled was achieved through legislative activity—as briefly surveyed above—court action was deemed an appropriate alternative.

The judicial origins of the "right to education" are based on the now-famous 1954 Supreme Court decision in *Brown* vs. *Board of Education* (Topeka, Kansas), which ruled that racially segregated schools were unconstitutional. The Court stated:

> In these days, it is doubtful that any child may reasonably be expected to succeed in life if he is denied the opportunity of an education. Such an opportunity, where the state has undertaken to provide it, is a right which must be made available to all on equal terms.[36]

The Supreme Court also stated in its ruling that "'separate but equal' is inherently unequal." This ruling has been applied to disabled children.

> . . . segregation . . . has a detrimental effect on exceptional children . . . the policy of separation . . . is usually interpreted as denoting the inferiority of exceptional groups; . . . the sense of inferiority affects motivation; segregation has the tendency to retard education and mental development of exceptional children and deprives them of benefits they would receive in totally integrated systems.[37]

Two key law suits established a right to due process protection in relation to educational classification or exclusion from publicly supported education systems. The PARC case, *Pennsylvania Association for Retarded Children* vs. *Pennsylvania* (1971), established for the first time that mentally retarded children, regardless of the severity of handicap, had the right to an appropriate educational opportunity at public expense.[38] It also stated that youngsters had the right to appeal the placement provided by the school system, if it was believed inappropriate. The *Mills* vs. *Board of Education* case (1972) ruled that all handicapped children, regardless of the disability, had a right to education.[39]

The "right to treatment" concept was probably first articulated by Dr. Martin Birnbaum in 1960, who attempted to focus public attention on the inadequacy of treatment for the mentally ill and suggested litigation that would remediate such inadequacies. The first suit involving disabled persons was that of *Wyatt* vs. *Stickney* (1972) in Alabama. This case established that persons confined against their will to public mental institutions and retardation facilities have a constitutional right to receive appropriate, individualized treatment. "Treatment" was defined in the case as a "realistic opportunity to lead a more useful and meaningful life and to return to society."[40] This case developed from a 1970s scenario in which filth and vermin prevailed in a hospital built in the mid-nineteenth century and which housed 5,000 residents. Straitjackets were often used and physical abuse was common. No specialists in retardation or geriatrics were on the staff. This gruesome picture was common in a majority of state hospitals in the U.S. at the time.

Other major rights that were addressed through the courts in the 1970s included "right to protection from harm," "right to refuse treatment," "right to fair compensation," "right to liberty," and "right to privacy," among others. The suits that brought attention to these human concerns were a result of intensive class-action efforts. Their effect has been not only to improve the quality of lives of people in institutional settings but also to point the direction in constitutional rights and social policy development.

One case, decided by a hearing officer in the Bureau of Special Appeals, Commonwealth of Massachusetts, in 1981, had implications for recreation. Known as the Tuttle case, the parents of a young girl with Down's syndrome were awarded a decision to include a therapeutic recreation program in their daughter's individual education plan (IEP). The school district was forced to hire a therapeutic recreator to provide services that focused on social skill development, decision making, development of knowledge about recreation, and leisure opportunities and activities. (Table 8-3 outlines major litigation cases.)

Beyond legislation and litigation, the recreation and leisure service profession has an ethical commitment to provide services to all persons regardless of age, race, sex, or ability. This commitment must be based on a solid understanding of ideologies underlying service provision.

The Age of Accountability

While efforts were being made to increase the opportunities available to persons with disabilities in educational, work, and community settings, therapeutic recreators working in clinical/medical settings were struggling

TABLE 8-3 Litigation: Significant Cases

YEAR	CASE	RULING
1954	Brown vs. Board of Education	"'Separate but equal' is inherently unequal"; black children are entitled to equal education
1971	PARC (Nancy Beth Bowman) vs. the Commonwealth of Pennsylvania	First established that mentally retarded children, regardless of severity of handicap, had the right to an appropriate educational opportunity at public expense
1972	Mills vs. Board of Education	All handicapped children have the right to education
1972	Wyatt vs. Stickney, Alabama	Individuals in public mental hospitals have a "right to treatment," including a humane physical and psychological environment; qualified staff in adequate numbers; individual treatment plan
1975	N.Y. State Association for Retarded Citizens vs. Carey, known as the Willowbrook case	Individuals in public institutions have a right to protection from harm

with the demands of a hospital and health care industry in transition. In the 1970s and continuing well into the 1980s, hospital costs soared. In order to contain these rising costs, many changes occurred, including the privatization of hospitals, the trend toward multihospital conglomerates, and efforts to reduce in-hospital service costs. A prospective-payment system was developed to reimburse hospitals according to predetermined prices based on classification of patients by diagnosis, age, needed medical procedures, and a standardized length of stay.[41] These classifications are termed *diagnostic related groups* (DRGs). As a result, all these changes had a dramatic impact on the provision of all health care services, including therapeutic recreation services.

Because personnel, facility space, equipment, and materials all cost money, therapeutic recreators were challenged to demonstrate that these costs benefitted the patient. Professionals had to document the efficacy of their services in order to survive.

While cost-benefit analysis was initially an issue in acute health care settings, it affects every setting in which services are provided. As consumers become more aware of their rights and the costs of services, they also demand effective service delivery from professionals.

An important part of the increased sophistication of the therapeutic recreation field is the need to account for how resources are used and the benefit that accrues from them. This issue will continue to occupy the attention of the profession in the future.

THE PROFESSIONAL AND PHILOSOPHICAL DEVELOPMENT OF THERAPEUTIC RECREATION

The development of therapeutic recreation has paralleled changes in broader social policies and national movements. Lee Meyer, past-president of the National Therapeutic Recreation Society (NTRS), presented a paper on the development of therapeutic recreation. The following section is derived from that paper. In this significant contribution, Dr. Meyer divides the profession's development into two broad time periods, the 1880s to the mid-1930s and the late 1930s to the mid-1960s.[42]

He refers to the earlier period as the "recreation in hospitals" era. In this phase, recreation activities were perceived as worthwhile diversions that redirected patients' energies and provided entertainment. Essentially, these programs were no different in intent from those programs in community settings. As voluntary, leisure-time activities, they were expected to elicit fun, relaxation, and enjoyment. Meyer notes that hospital and community recreation programs represented distinct efforts, because there was no professional entity responsible for recreation at the time. He characterizes this period in the following way:

1. The provision of recreational opportunities was the focus of recreation programs for ill and disabled, both in hospitals and community settings.
2. Recreation in hospitals had its beginning separate from the community-focused play/recreation movement.
3. Efforts to provide recreational opportunities for disabled children in community settings were contemporary with, but independent from, recreation in hospitals.
4. The service characteristics of recreational programs were essentially the same for recreation in hospitals, recreation for disabled children in community settings, and for the community-based recreation movement at the time.
5. Although separate origins seem evident, the nature and purpose of recreation services were essentially the same, differing only in regard to the setting in which services were provided and/or the intended recipients of the services.[43]

The beginning of the professional period, from the late 1930s to the mid-1960s, saw the development of three philosophical orientations. The first two, which Meyers terms "hospital recreation" and "recreation therapy," were hospital-based. The third, "recreation for the ill and handicapped," was community-based.

Both the hospital recreation and recreation for ill and handicapped (community-based) perspectives emphasized the tenet that recreation is a wholesome endeavor, contributing to physical, social, mental, and emotional well-being. David Gray characterizes what has been termed "the recreative experience" in what is now a classical quote.

> Recreation is an emotional condition within an individual human being that flows from a feeling of well-being and satisfaction. It is characterized by feelings of mastery, achievement, exhilaration, acceptance, success, personal worth, and pleasure. It reinforces a positive self-image. Recreation is a response to an esthetic experience, an achievement of personal goals or positive feedback from others. It is independent of activity, leisure, or social acceptance.[44]

The recreative experience was perceived to have therapeutic benefits. That is, it contributed to a positive psychological state by increasing one's confidence and self-esteem, and it was a factor in personal growth and development. Its primary aim was to enhance individual feelings of satisfaction and enjoyment.

Hospital recreation was seen as an area of specialization within the emerging recreation movement. Its goals were not seen as different from organized recreation services provided within the community.

The third perspective, termed *recreation therapy*, took a very different approach. It was characterized by the following:

1. Recreation activities were considered to effect treatment goals;
2. Recreation activities were used for therapy, with secondary emphasis on enjoyment;

3. The providers of recreation therapy saw themselves as therapists; they had little identification with the organized recreation movement;
4. The therapists were primarily concerned with the treatment of disease.[45]

The "recreation versus therapy" philosophical conflict resulted in the establishment of two organizations—the Hospital Section of the American Recreation Society, and the National Association of Recreation Therapists.

The term *therapeutic recreation* was first used by Beatrice Hill in 1957 to refer to specialized recreation services for hospitalized and the noninstitutionalized ill and handicapped.[46] This concept was seen as an extension of the "recreation for all" principle and introduced the recreation worker as a new member of the team in specialized areas.[47] Meyers notes:

> Therapeutic recreation from its introduction in this 1957 article represented a seemingly intended unification of previously separate concerns: hospital recreation (recreation in hospitals) and recreation for the ill and handicapped in the community; that is, recreation services for the noninstitutionalized ill and handicapped.[48]

This dual emphasis parallels the early transition of ill and disabled individuals from institutional to community settings.

In 1966, the divergent perspectives were unified through the formation of the National Therapeutic Recreation Society (NTRS) as a branch of the National Recreation and Park Association (NRPA). Since that time, the term *therapeutic recreation* has come to be the principal designation of specialized recreation services for persons with illnesses and disabilities. The term serves as an umbrella for, and unification of, the perspectives identified above. However, controversy and discussion abound on what term or label best reflects the profession and what the profession should encompass.

In 1981, the membership of NTRS voted on three philosophical positions presented by Meyers, based upon his extensive review of the literature. The membership was asked to select which of the following perspectives best represented the field and which should be the concern of NTRS.

Position 1: The Continuum Model (Gunn and Peterson)

The purpose of therapeutic recreation from this perspective is "to provide treatment to those persons who have been determined to be in need of it, and/or provide opportunities for recreation to those persons needing special programmatic adaptations which facilitate recreation participation, irrespective of the setting in which these services are provided."[49]

Position 2: The Recreation Perspective

This perspective represents those who "provide opportunities for recreation to those persons needing special programmatic adaptations which facilitate recreational participation." In this position, therapeutic recreation would be synonymous with special recreation or recreation for special populations.

Position 3: The Treatment Perspective

This perspective represents those who provide treatment (health restoration, remediation, habilitation, rehabilitation, etc.) to those persons who have been determined to be in need of it, irrespective of the setting in which the service is provided.[50]

While only a small percentage of the membership voted, it selected the continuum orientation as the favored perspective. This perspective was based on the Peterson and Gunn model (refer to Chapter 3).

A philosophical position statement was then developed by NTRS, which further explained this model. This statement is included at the end of the chapter. The reader who is interested in a more detailed description of philosophical positions and their implications should refer to the paper by Meyer.

New Professional Directions

In 1984, the American Therapeutic Recreation Association (ATRA) was formed in response to the needs of professionals primarily working in health and human-care facilities. Independent of other therapeutic recreation or leisure-service organizations, this association emphasized the treatment and education (intervention-oriented) functions of the field. ATRA's stated aim was to respond to the need for accountability facing the therapeutic recreation profession.[51]

The development of this organization 18 years after the establishment of NTRS was a reflection of the continuing changes in the field and in society at large. Along with the evolution of society, we can expect the therapeutic recreation profession to also undergo evolution. Some of the issues that will continue confronting the profession are addressed in Chapter 14.

SUMMARY

This chapter summarized the evolution of services to ill and disabled persons, including therapeutic recreation services from the beginnings of early history to the present. This development was characterized within the social and cultural milieu of each era. The change in the orientation of services was shown to be from maintenance and custodial services, to treatment of illness and disability, to education, and to the integration of persons with disabilities into the mainstream of society. Although the status of persons with disabilities has not yet reached an acceptable level, we can be encouraged by the tremendous changes that have occurred over the last 20 years.

The chapter ended with a review of the development of the therapeutic recreation field from the later part of the nineteenth century to the present. The currently accepted philosophical position of NTRS encompasses a range of services from therapy to recreation. It has been suggested that the philosophy will continue to evolve as professionals challenge their own views in a rapidly changing society. Further, as our profession develops, therapeutic recreators will continue to ask how we can further contribute to society's acceptance of people with disabilities.

NATIONAL RECREATION AND PARK ASSOCIATION

PHILOSOPHICAL POSITION STATEMENT
OF THE
NATIONAL THERAPEUTIC RECREATION SOCIETY

(A Branch of the National Recreation and Park Association)

(Adopted, May 1982)

Lesiure, including recreation and play, are inherent aspects of the human experience. The importance of appropriate leisure involvement has been documented throughout history. More recently, research has addressed the value of leisure involvement in human development, in social and family relationships, and in general, as an important aspect of the quality of life. Some human beings have disabilities, illnesses, or social conditions which limit their full participation in the normative social structure of society. These individuals with limitations have the same human rights to, and needs for, leisure involvement.

The purpose of therapeutic recreation is to facilitate the development, maintenance, and expression of an appropriate leisure lifestyle for individuals with physical, mental, emotional, or social limitations. Accordingly, this purpose is accomplished through the provision of professional programs and services which assist the client in eliminating barriers to leisure, developing leisure skills and attitudes, and optimizing leisure involvement. Therapeutic-recreation professionals use these principles to enhance clients' leisure ability in recognition of the importance and value of leisure in the human experience.

Three specific areas of professional services are employed to provide this comprehensive leisure ability approach toward enabling appropriate leisure lifestyles: therapy, leisure education, and recreation participation. While these three areas of service have unique purposes in relation to client need, they each employ similar delivery processes using assessment or identification of client need, development of a related program strategy, and monitoring and evaluating client outcomes. The decision as to where and when each of the three service areas would be provided is based on the assessment of client needs and the service mandate of the sponsoring agency. The selection of appropriate service areas is contingent on a recognition that different clients have differing needs related to leisure involvement in view of their personal life situation.

The purpose of the *therapy* service area within therapeutic recreation is to improve functional behaviors. Some clients may require treatment or remediation of a functional behavior as a necessary prerequisite to enable their involvement in meaningful leisure experiences. *Therapy*, therefore, is viewed as most appropriate when clients have functional limitations that relate to, or inhibit, their potential leisure involvement. This distinction enables the therapeutic recreator to decide when *therapy* service is appropriate, as well as to identify the types of behaviors that are most appropriate to address within the therapeutic recreation domain of expertise and authority. In settings where a comprehensive treatment team approach is used, *therapy* focuses on team identified treatment goals, as well as addressing unique aspects of leisure related functional behaviors. This approach places therapeutic recreation as an integral and cooperative member of the comprehensive treatment team, while linking its primary focus to eventual leisure ability.

The purpose of the *leisure education* service area is to provide opportunities for the acquisition of skills, knowledge, and attitudes related to leisure involvement. For some clients, acquiring leisure skills, knowledge, and attitudes are priority needs. It appears that the majority of clients in residential, treatment, and community settings need *leisure education* services in order to initiate and engage in leisure experiences. It is the absence of leisure learning opportunities and socialization into leisure that blocks or inhibits these individuals from participation in leisure experiences. Here, *leisure education* services would be employed to provide the client with leisure skills, enhance the client's attitudes concerning the value and importance of leisure, as well as learning about opportunities and resources for leisure involvement. Thus, *leisure education* programs provide the opportunity for the development of leisure behaviors and skills.

The purpose of the *recreation participation* area of therapeutic recreation services is to provide opportunities which allow voluntary client involvement in recreation interests and activities. Human beings, despite disability, illness, or other limiting conditions, and, regardless of place of residence, are entitled to recreation opportunities. The justification for specialized *recreation participation* programs is based on the clients' need for assistance and/or adapted recreation equipment, limitations imposed by restrictive treatment or residential environments, or the absence of appropriate community recreation opportunities. In therapeutic recreation services, the need for *recreation participation* is acknowledged and given appropriate emphasis in recognition of the intent of the leisure ability concept.

These three service areas of therapeutic recreation represent a continuum of care, including *therapy, leisure education,* and the provision of special *recreation participation* opportunities. This comprehensive leisure ability approach uses the need of the client to give direction to program service selection. In some situations, the client may need programs from all three service areas. In other situations, the client may require only one or two of the service areas.

Equally important is the concern of generalizing therapeutic-recreation service across diverse service delivery settings. The leisure ability approach of therapeutic recreation provides appropriate program direction regardless of type of setting or type of client served. A professional working in a treatment setting can see the extension of the leisure ability approach toward client needs within the community environment. Likewise, those within the community can view therapeutic recreation services within a perspective of previous services received or possible future needs.

All human beings, including those individuals with disabilities, illnesses, or limiting conditions, have a right to, and a need for, leisure involvement as a necessary aspect of the human experience. The purpose of therapeutic recreation services is to facilitate the development, maintenance, and expression of an appropriate leisure lifestyle for individuals with limitations through the provision of *therapy, leisure education,* and *recreation participation* services.

The National Therapeutic Recreation Society is the acknowledged professional organization representing the field of therapeutic recreation. The National Therapeutic Recreation Society exists to foster the development and advancement of this field in order to ensure quality professional services and to protect the rights of consumers of therapeutic recreation services. In order to provide consistent and identifiable services throughout the field, the National Therapeutic Recreation Society endorses the leisure ability philosophy described herein as the official position statement regarding therapeutic recreation.

DISCUSSION QUESTIONS

8-1.   The evolution of therapeutic recreation reflects the evolution of society. Succinctly, characterize (1) the nature of society, (2) how leisure and (3) disability were viewed, and (4) the status of rehabilitation in the major eras:

	SOCIETY	LEISURE	DISABILITY	REHABILI-TATION
Folk era				
Agrarian society				
Greek and Roman civilizations				
Middle Ages (effect of Christianity)				
Reformation/ Renaissance				
Colonial America				
Industrialism mid-nineteenth century				
Turn of the century				
1960s and 1970s				

8–2. What was the role of legislation and litigation in ensuring the rights of persons with disabilities?

8–3. Think of the major national or international social events and trends (political, economic, demographic) that have happened in your own lifetime and list them. Can you identify ways in which your life, or that of your family or members of your community, was influenced by these events? (For example, has the onset of the "Communications/Computer/Technology Age" influenced the way you live?) Can you explain how therapeutic recreation services are a reflection of what happened or is happening in society? Why is it important to be alert to major national and international events or trends occurring in society?

8–4. The therapeutic recreation service model (the continuum) provides one basis for the way that therapeutic recreation is viewed. You will see reference to it time and time again. Explain the continuum. The NTRS Philosophical Position Statement reprinted at the end of this chapter explains the continuum. What is meant by *leisure-ability*? Explain.

NOTES

[1]Johan Huizinga, *Homo Ludens: A Study of the Play Elements in Culture* (Boston: Beacon Press, 1950); Virginia Frye and Martha Peters, *Therapeutic Recreation: Its Theory, Philosophy and Practice* (Harrisburg, Penn.: Stackpole Books, 1972); John Kelly, *Leisure* (Englewood Cliffs, N.J.: Prentice-Hall, 1982).

[2]Huizinga, *Homo Ludens.*

[3]Ronald Adams, Alfred N. Daniel, and Lee Rullman, *Games, Sports and Exercises for the Physically Handicapped* (Philadelphia: Lee & Febiger, 1972), p. 5.

[4]Ibid.

[5]Frye and Peters, *Therapeutic Recreation,* pp. 16–17.

[6]Ibid., p. 17.

[7]Gerald O'Morrow, *Therapeutic Recreation: A Helping Profession,* 2nd ed. (Reston, Va.: Reston Publishing Co., 1980), p. 88.

[8]Ibid., p. 88.

[9]John Lenihan, *Performance, Disabled Americans: A History,* President's Committee on the Employment of the Handicapped, XXVII, 5-6-7 (1976–77), p. 5.

[10]Ibid.

[11]Ibid.

[12]Ibid.

[13]Robert M. Goldenson, ed., *Disability and Rehabilitation Handbook* (San Francisco: McGraw-Hill, 1978), p. 4.

[14]Lenihan, *Performance, Disabled Americans,* p. 8.

[15]Ibid., p. 12.

[16]Ibid., pp. 15–18.

[17]Ibid., p. 20.

[18]Ibid., p. 19.

[19]Ibid., pp. 19–20.

[20]Ibid., p. 21.

[21]Goldenson, *Disability and Rehabilitation,* p. 4.

[22]O'Morrow, *Therapeutic Recreation,* p. 97.

[23]Richard Kraus, *Therapeutic Recreation Service: Principles and Practices,* 3rd ed. (Philadelphia: Saunders, 1983), p. 25.

[24]Thomas A. Stein and Douglas Sessoms, *Recreation and Special Populations,* 2nd ed. (Boston: Holbrook Press, 1983), p. 4.

[25]Adams and others, *Games, Sports and Exercises,* pp. 8–9.

[26]American Coalition of Citizens with Disabilities, Inc., Pamphlet, Washington, D.C., n.d.

[27]"National Forum on Meeting the Recreation and Park Needs of Handicapped People," President's Committee on Employment of the Handicapped, Washington, D.C., NRPA, 1974, p. 5.

[28]Frederick Fay and Janet Minch, *Access to Recreation: A Report on the National Hearing for Handicapped Persons,* HEW: Office of Human Development and Rehabilitation Services Administration, 1977, pp. 53–62.

[29]*Awareness Papers,* White House Conference on Handicapped Individuals, 1977, p. v.

[30]*Final Report,* White House Conference on Handicapped Individuals, 1977, pp. 78–84.

[31]Stephen Klement, "Removing Architectural Barriers," in Goldenson, *Disability and Rehabilitation,* p. 111.

[32]Architectural and Transportation Barriers Act of 1968, P.L. 90–480.

[33]Section 504, 1973 Rehabilitation Act, P.L. 93–112.

[34]Roxanne Howe-Murphy, "The Identification of Guidelines for Mainstreaming Recreation and Leisure Services" (unpublished Master's thesis, San Jose State University, 1978), pp. 109–111, 119.

[35]William Dussault, "Legislation and Consumer Rights: Federal and State Laws," in Goldenson, *Disability and Rehabilitation,* pp. 127–136; David Park, *Legislation Affecting Park Services and Recreation for Handicapped Individuals* (Washington, D.C.: Hawkins and Associates, 1980); Jerry Kelley, ed., *Recreation Programming for Visually Impaired Children and Youth* (New York: American Foundation for the Blind, 1981), pp. 3–4; Lee Meyer, "Recreation and the Mentally Ill," in Stein and Sessoms, *Recreation and Special Populations,* pp. 154–155.

[36]*Brown* vs. *Board of Education,* Topeka, Kansas, 1954.

[37]Florence Christoplos and Paul Renz, "A Critical Examination of Special Education Programs," *The Journal of Special Education,* 3 (1969), 377.

[38]Dussault, "Legislation and Consumer

Rights," in Goldenson, *Disability and Rehabilitation*, p. 129.

[39]Ibid.

[40]Lee A. Carty, "Advocacy," in Goldenson, *Disability and Rehabilitation*, p. 147.

[41]Mary S. Reitter, "Third Party Reimbursement: Is Therapeutic Recreation Too Late?" *Therapeutic Recreation Journal*, 4 (1984), 14.

[42]Lee Meyer, *Philosophical Alternatives and the Professionalization of Therapeutic Recreation* (Chapel Hill: University of North Carolina Press, 1980), pp. 4–36.

[43]Ibid., pp. 5–6.

[44]David Gray, "Exploring Inner Space," *Parks and Recreation*, 7 (1972), p. 19.

[45]Meyer, "Philosophical Alternatives," pp. 9–10.

[46]Ibid., p. 11.

[47]Ibid., p. 12.

[48]Ibid.

[49]Scout Gunn and Carol Ann Peterson, *Therapeutic Recreation Program Design: Principles and Procedures* (Englewood Cliffs, N.J.: Prentice Hall, 1978), p. 33.

[50]Meyer, pp. 40, 42, 43.

[51]American Therapeutic Recreation Association, *ATRA Newsletter* (Stillwater, Okla., 1984).

9

CONTEMPORARY CORNERSTONES OF SERVICE DELIVERY

Members of the therapeutic recreation course assembled for a debriefing shortly after field trips they had taken. The instructor had suggested that, as a group, they visit the state school for mentally retarded persons not far from the college and, individually, visit one of the nursing homes in the vicinity. "Let's talk about what you saw, heard and smelled—and how you feel about the places you visited."

Deanna blurted out, "I was terrified about going, because I had only heard stories about those places. I had never been to one before. I didn't like it at all. The smells. . . . "

Maria: "I didn't think the school was so bad. I was surprised that the residents could do so much, like take care of their rooms and go to different buildings on the campus without help. But I was wondering why they were living there instead of somewhere else. I guess that there aren't many good living alternatives available for people."

Renee: "Did you see the way some of them were dressed? They would never be accepted in the community looking that way. Besides, they acted sort of different—maybe they really can't do any more without constant supervision."

Robert: "The nursing home that I saw was the pits. Poeple were just sitting around; there was no life in the place. The residents all looked ready to die. My grandmother used to live in a nursing home, a good one. She shared a room, but got to decorate part of it with her things. She often participated in activities that she enjoyed. And the place had life. The staff was terrific—very caring and provided a lot of freedom to the residents."

"You obviously have a lot of reactions to your observations," said the instructor. "And you're noticing important factors in the environment that help the people in the environment maintain or lose their dignity. You already have a sense that the nature of the environment has a lot to do with the way we perceive the people. Let's continue."

INTRODUCTION

Earlier in this book we reviewed the evolution of therapeutic recreation services. We explored briefly the nature of leisure and play—and what these phenomena mean to people. We also discussed the relationship of health and well-being to leisure behavior. In essence, we were talking about some of the *content* of human experience.

In this chapter, we will delve into the *structure* of experiences provided by therapeutic recreators. The way in which services are designed is critical to how the consumer perceives the experience.

Of course, structure should not be thought of as being static. Programs and services should be designed to be responsive to the people served. This chapter provides some guidelines and a context for designing effective supportive services.

NORMALIZATION

The principle of *normalization* has evolved as an internationally influential paradigm serving as a cornerstone for human-service delivery systems for all persons with disabilities.[1] Initially introduced in Denmark by Bank-Mikkelson to govern services for mentally retarded persons in the 1950s, it has since come to have broader implications. Wolfensberger provided the first comprehensive interpretation of the concept of normalization:

> . . . the utilization of means which are culturally as normative as possible in order to establish, enable or support behaviors, appearances, experiences, and interpretations which are as culturally normative as possible.[2]

This definition emphasizes both the *means* (process) and the *ends* (outcome) that ultimately offer life conditions which are culturally valued to persons with disabilities. Confusion surrounds the term because some people have isolated the word "normal" and erroneously interpreted it to mean that disabled persons should be "rendered normal." More correctly, it does mean making housing, education, employment, and leisure conditions as typical as possible. These, in turn, elicit images and behaviors that are valued and supported by society.

The Power of Imagery

Central to the methods utilized and outcomes evoked is the issue of *imagery*. What is the message given to the disabled individual or given to the public when disabled persons are treated differently and are separated from the remainder of society? The normalization principle implies that each person is entitled to be presented in as positive a manner as possible.

Consider, if you will, the personal and social effects of the following: being called a retarded person; of going to a facility located next to other facilities that serve only other persons with disabilities; of being treated as a child, even though you are an adult; of being given meaningless work and play activities to do. Every action that service providers take, every decision about how services will be delivered, and the terms used to refer to programs and to clients—all have inherent messages about the consumer. Too often the messages, consciously or unconsciously, imply deviance, a negative value in society. And consumers are generally just as aware of these messages and images about them as the rest of society.

If we see an adult who is disabled, wears clothes that are too large, has a "bowl" haircut, and attends a summer camp called "Sunnyside," our perception of that person is apt to be negatively affected. We are likely to interpret these perceptions as indicating that the individual is not competent. Conversely, images can also have the opposite effect; that is, to *enhance* perceptions of individuals. The way in which we address people is an example. An adult male who is called Bill may receive more positive recognition than if he is called "Billy," which carries with it a childlike connotation.

Images, then, can either enhance or degrade. On a personal level, images are derived from titles, names, or labels; from clothing worn; from haircuts and the condition of one's teeth, among other indicators. On a program/activity/facility level, images are formed through titles or labels; through the actual activity and its appropriateness to age; and through the way the activity is conducted.

Signals or cues in the environment or on the person that elicit negative attention or produce instant recognition of some oddity (deviance) may be called "clangers."[3] Clangers include out-of-style haircuts, out-of-style clothes, and unkempt appearances. Of course, some individuals choose to dress outrageously for the purpose of attracting attention. What we are discussing here is not so much a matter of educated option, but of the *only* option. Other clangers include adults playing games associated with childhood; again, not from a matter of choice, but as the only activity provided.

Of what importance are clangers to therapeutic recreators and other leisure-service personnel? First, we are all apt to be faced with individuals who appear to be deviant. How do we react to these individuals? Human nature being what it is, we just might forget that the individual indeed appears more deviant because of his or her clothes, the activities in which he or she is engaging, or the title of the program that the person is attending.

Let us not forget that the image is not necessarily reflective of who the person is and what the person can do. Frankly, there may be little we can personally do to eliminate the clanger itself. If an adult is attending the Crippled Children's camp, we may have no power to change the name of the camp or agency.

On the other hand, there are some clangers that we, as people and as professional service providers, can eliminate or minimize. We can ensure that our interactions with persons who are disabled reflect respect and dignity of that person. We can deliver programs that emphasize skills, abilities, and strengths of people, rather than those that emphasize the disability. Would *you* rather attend a Sports Program that can be adapted to meet individual needs or a Handicapped Sports Program?

Why should we be so concerned with names and titles? For one thing, we all know that words carry with them powerful connotations and perceptions. There is ample evidence to indicate that our perceptions lead to expectations. And there is the self-fulfilling prophecy that suggests the potency of our expectations: We tend to fulfill our expectations.

If a person is perceived as being "very different," not only because of visible physical traits but also because of clothing or the environment in which he or she lives, works, or plays, it is likely that not much will be expected from that person behaviorally. Rather, deviant behaviors are often tolerated, below-average achievement at work, school, or home is allowed to continue, and inappropriate social interactions persist. Frequently, these behaviors serve to further isolate the individual from others. Thus, the self-fulfilling prophecy manifests itself successfully.

Service providers must ensure that they don't get caught in and perpetuate the cycle of disability and deviance. Rather, if you believe that people with disabilities can and will grow, learn, and develop, then the methods (strategies for providing programs and opportunities) that you select will most likely succeed in fulfilling *that* expectation.

If we wholeheartedly believe that mentally retarded persons can successfully interact in a social situation, we are prone to teach and demand the requisite skills. If, however, we think that these individuals probably cannot attain an appropriate social level of functioning, we might tend to allow behaviors that are disruptive or overly affectionate. For example, people typically do not approach strangers they meet with a hug and kiss. Often, however, one may observe a young adult with Down's syndrome constantly hugging people. While this behavior may be appropriate on occasion, it is not generally acceptable. A professional who expects an individual to interact appropriately in social settings will not permit continuation of that or similar behavior. Instead, substitute behaviors, such as a handshake and verbal greeting, will be taught.

This concept of normalization and the power of imagery is closely connected to attribution theory, discussed earlier in the text. Through the use of normalized environments, both actors (consumers) and observers (service personnel, able-bodied peers, and others) are more likely to attribute competence to the actor.

Selected Components of Normalization

Nirje, an early proponent and interpreter of the normalization principle, outlined several components that help explain how to put the concept into operation.[4]

1. Normal Rhythm of the Day

A normalized rhythm of day refers to one's right to engage in meaningful daily activities in a normal fashion.

2. Normal Rhythm of the Week

This refers to one's right to engage in a variety of meaningful life experiences, including work, education and leisure.

3. Normal Rhythm of the Year

This principle refers to the right of everyone to have typical experiences reflective of yearly patterns.

4. Normal Experiences of the Life Cycle

The opportunities to experience the normal developmental phases of life are central to maturing as an individual. This principle, then, is based upon each individual's right to have access to age-appropriate experiences.

5. Normal Respect

The interests, wishes, and desires of persons with disabilities must not only be considered, but elicited. For those who are nonverbal or who have difficulty in communicating, this central concept becomes even a bigger challenge. Personal preferences in hairstyle, clothing, activities, personal environment and social networks should all be recognized, regardless of one's level of disability.

6. Living in a Heterosexual World

The integration of sexes, representing typical social patterns in everyday life, can be expected to improve behavior and minimize unnecessary loneliness.

7. Normal Economic Standards

An acceptable financial level increases one's personal access to a realm of opportunities as well as enhances self-concept.

8. Normal Environmental Standards

Specialized physical facilities such as schools, leisure settings, work sites, and homes (such as group homes) should be modeled after those available to the community at large.

The eight components of normalization that we have just enumerated may seem to be "common sense." "Of course!" you say indignantly. "These are basic human rights!" These principles remind us how much we each take for granted when we recognize that many of these basic rights have been denied to large groups of ill, elderly, and disabled persons. Remember, Nirje first delineated these rights in the 1960s in response to their absence.

Before proceeding, take some time to complete the exercise outlined in Table 9–1, excerpted from *The Normalization Folio*.[5] The exercise reminds

TABLE 9–1
INDIVIDUAL RIGHTS

Read through the following list of human rights. If you are tempted to view these pronouncements as platitudes with only limited significance to yourself, try this exercise: List the three rights that you would be willing to sacrifice if you had to cut your list to 10. You have *no* choice. You *must* give up three! Which three?

-Love, honor, and freedom from stigma throughout life
-The celebration of being special
-A life-sharing family, home, and nurturing support
-A community of concern and friendship
-Economic security, health, and the full benefits of modern technology, with a full continuum of services
-Freedom from the threat of injury due to pollution of food, air, water, and the earth on which we dwell
-The opportunity to grow, learn, choose, work, rest, play, be nourished, and to experience well-being
-Solitude when needed
-Space, comfort, and beauty to discover one's self
-The power to improve one's personal environment
-Justice
-The dignity of risk, joy, and the growth of spirit
-A valued social future

Now, cut your list to seven (of the original 13). Which three rights would you give up next?

How many rights can you cross off your list before you begin to feel dehumanized? If people who have special needs do not have these rights, are they, then, dehumanized? How can you tell?

us that what we often take for granted is not always available to everyone—without a fight.

Largely as a result of the confusion surrounding the term *normalization,* practitioners have experienced difficulty in bringing the theory into practice. While it is the authors' intent to reflect this principle in discussion of professional practices throughout the text, some basic applications are outlined here.

Wolfensberger proposed several corollaries, or intricately related concepts, to normalization in his 1972 text.[6] They are identified in Table 9–2. Review them carefully, as they are critical to understanding normalization. The material can be used to evaluate programs, settings, and activities serving individuals with disabilities.

Hutchison and Lord, in an important contribution to the field, pro-

TABLE 9-2 Major Corollaries of Normalization: How Do Services Rate?

BRIEF DESCRIPTION 1. PHYSICAL INTEGRATION	YES	NO
Physical integration allows for physical proximity of non-disabled and disabled persons. This basic level of integration is determined by several characteristics of the environment (i.e., facilities used for services and programs):		
(a) Geographical proximity of a program or service facility: Is the facility in an area that is geographically accessible?	————	————
(b) Transportation: Is the facility used accessible by some convenient form of transportation (i.e., accessible public transportation, wheelchair, accessible vans, carpools)?	————	————
(c) Neighborhood characteristics: Does the neighborhood housing the facility support community resources such as stores and service centers?	————	————
(d) Facility size: Is the facility small enough to be an integral and accepted part of the neighborhood?	————	————
2. SOCIAL INTEGRATION		
Social integration is the interaction of disabled and non-disabled persons. This more complex level of integration is determined by several characteristics:		
(a) Design of the program: Does it encourage the involvement of nondisabled and disabled persons?	————	————
(b) Program and consumer terminology: Are terms used that stress the purpose of the program and that reflect the total person?	————	————
(c) Facility esthetics: Is the facility used attractive, desirable, and esthetically pleasing?	————	————

(continued)

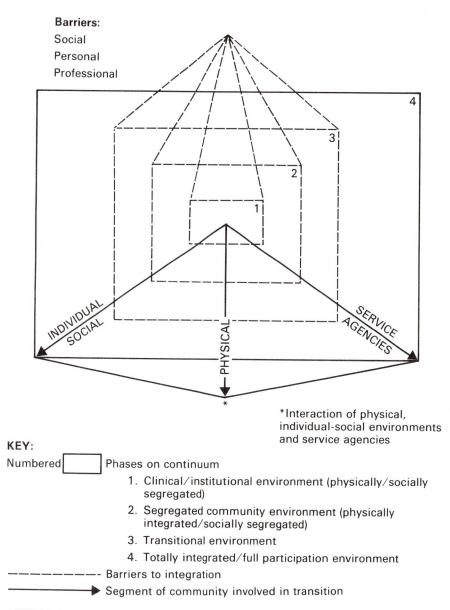

Barriers:
Social
Personal
Professional

*Interaction of physical, individual-social environments and service agencies

KEY:
Numbered ☐ Phases on continuum

1. Clinical/institutional environment (physically/socially segregated)
2. Segregated community environment (physically integrated/socially segregated)
3. Transitional environment
4. Totally integrated/full participation environment

——————— Barriers to integration
——————▶ Segment of community involved in transition

FIGURE 9-2   An Ecological Mainstreaming Model. Adapted from J. Spinak, *Leisurability*, 2, 1975.

in designing services but increases our understanding that success or failure lies not in the individual with the disability.

A synthesis of the principles of mainstreaming and their implications are listed in Table 9-5.

TABLE 9-5 A Synthesis: Mainstreaming Principles

PRINCIPLE OF MAINSTREAMING	IMPLICATION OF PRINCIPLE

1. Recognition of the individual	1. Individualization of service
	    continuum of services responding to
	    intraindividual differences
	    changes in person over period of time

2. Respect for the individual	2. Multiplicity of roles for disabled person
	    recipient of services
	    source of knowledge, resources
	    participant in planning, providing, and evaluating service
	    independent decision-maker
	    advisor

3. Twofold process	3. Skill-development opportunities for all individuals
	    community education
	    role versatility for therapeutic and general recreators

4. "Mainstreaming the system"	4. Changes within the system of services
	    training/retraining of staff
	    facilities accessible
	    progams accessible
	    involvement of disabled and non-disabled participants together
	    education of parents
	    education of community
	    interagency cooperation

5. Continuum of services	5. linkage among programs
	    interagency cooperation
	    support services
	    assessment and evaluation of services

SUMMARY

This chapter discussed two basic foundations for the design of leisure and therapeutic recreation services. *Normalization* refers to both the means and goal of providing culturally typical environments and expectations to persons who are disabled. *Imagery*, which is created through services, provokes perceptions about persons and can serve to dignify or dehumanize the consumer.

Mainstreaming refers to multiple processes that maximize individual ability and minimize the effects of barriers to one's full participation in life's opportunities. Several variables were identified that contribute to the success of mainstreaming efforts; therefore, the term *mainstreaming the system* was used. This concept and its applications have potential benefits for all individuals, not just those with disabilities.

DISCUSSION QUESTIONS

9-1. Define *normalization* in your own words.

9-2. Discuss the power of *imagery.*

9-3. Complete Figure 9-1 included in the chapter.

9-4. List five "clangers" that you notice in society in general that give us messages about people with disabilities. These could be images in the physical environment, from the media, or from any other source. What negative messages about people with disabilities do you remember from childhood books?

9-5. List five positive messages about people with disabilities that you notice in society in general. Use the same sources as suggested above, if appropriate.

9-6. Define *mainstreaming* in your own words.

9-7. What are the four phases of the mainstreaming continuum? What is the purpose of each?

9-8. Distinguish between *physical* and *social* integration.

CASE STUDY

Four or five students will work as a unit for this activity. The group will select a therapeutic recreation program category serving a specific population that is vulnerable to the effects of "clangers." You may select from the following: (1) a nursing home for ill, elderly persons; (2) a residential school for children and youth with mental retardation; (3) a community recreation program serving primarily mentally retarded adults; or (4) another category of your choice. It will be helpful to select a category that everyone in the group has familiarity with either from personal experience or which can be gained from visits to sites within your community.

Part I

The first part of this activity may need to take place between class meetings. Visit a real-life example of the kind of setting you have selected. (Or recall the nature of the setting from your past experience. If you are involved in a field-work experience, perhaps you could use this as a setting.) Group members are urged to visit different facilities that reflect your category, in order to gather more information that will be helpful in proceeding with Part II. Be sure to make arrangements for this visit in advance with the appropriate person. Before the actual visit, review Table 9–2 carefully. During the visit, make mental notes on how the therapeutic recreation program does or does not reflect the corollaries of normalization. Does anything stand out as a "clanger"? Recall the questions posed earlier in the chapter: Are the conditions that you observe acceptable for you? Are they appropriate? The purpose of this visit is not to be critical of existing services, but rather to examine ways in which we often nonintentionally violate human dignity and to note ways in which people's human rights are carefully protected.

Discuss your observations with your group. Make a list entitled "Clangers." Write everything you believe fits under this category. Make a separate list, entitled "Positive Messages." Again, write down everything you believe fits into this category from your combined observations. Discuss these in class.

Part II

As a therapeutic recreation staff, your group is responsible for designing a program within this setting, which is based upon the principles of normalization. Be realistic in the decisions you make. For example, you will not have the power within the organization to build a new facility in order to have it close to community transportation. On the other hand, perhaps you can think of ways to find alternate modes of transportation that will help residents get into the community more often. Or, you may not have the power to change the name of the organization, but you can change the name of your program, if it is a "clanger." It may help to break your design into the five sections listed on Table 9–1: physical integration, social integration, right to self-determination, dignity of risk, and age-appropriate experiences. Perhaps you will want to add other categories.

Share your design with the remainder of the class. What difficulties did you encounter in trying to design a normalization-based program?

NOTES

[1]Robert J. Flynn and Kathleen Nitsch, eds., "The Normalization Principle: Systematic Statements and Clarifications," in *Normalization, Social Integration and Community Services* (Baltimore: University Park Press, 1980), p. 3.

[2]Wolf Wolfensberger, *The Principle of Normalization in Human Services* (Toronto: National Institute on Mental Retardation, 1972), p. 29.

[3]California State University and College Board of Trustees, "Normalization Folio," *Way to Go Series* (Baltimore: University Park Press, 1978), p. 25.

[4]Bengt Nirje, "The Normalization Principle," in *Normalization, Social Integration and Community Services*, eds. Robert J. Flynn and Kathleen E. Nitsch (Baltimore: University Park Press, 1980), pp. 36–44.

[5]California State University and Col-

lege Board of Trustees, "Normalization Folio," p. 50.

⁶Wolfensberger, *Normalization.*

⁷California State University and College Board of Trustees, "Normalization Folio," p. 29.

⁸Geoffrey Godbey, "Planning for Leisure in a Pluralistic Society," in *Recreation and Leisure Issues: An Era of Change,* eds. Thomas L. Goodale and Peter A. Witt (State College, Penn.: Venture, 1980), pp. 165–174.

⁹Michael F. Hogan, "Normalization and Communitization" in Flynn and Nitsch, *Normalization, Social Integration and Community Services,* pp. 299–312.

¹⁰M. Santamour and K. Rose, "Defining the Problem of Mental Retardation: A Functional Model." Paper presented at the Region X AAMD Meeting, 1969, in William A. Ayres, "Application of Technology and Rehabilitation Engineering, Part A: The Application of Technology to Handicapping Conditions and for Handicapped Individuals," *White House Conference on Handicapped Individuals Awareness Papers,* Washington, D.C., 1977, p. 25.

¹¹James F. Murphy, *Recreation and Leisure Services: A Humanistic Perspective* (Dubuque, Ia.: Wm. C. Brown, 1975), p. 2.

¹²Roxanne Howe-Murphy, "A Conceptual Basis for Mainstreaming Recreation and Leisure Services: Focus on Humanism," *Therapeutic Recreation Journal* XIII, 4 (1979), 13.

¹³William Gardner, *Learning and Behavioral Characteristics of Exceptional Children and Youth: A Humanistic Behavioral Approach* (Boston: Allyn & Bacon, 1977), p. 53.

¹⁴G. W. Allport, *Patterns and Growth on Personality* (New York: Holt, Rinehart & Winston, 1961).

¹⁵E.A. Doll, "Retrospect and Prospect," *Educating Trainable Mentally Retarded,* 1 (1966), 7.

¹⁶Florence Christopolos and Paul Renz, "A Critical Examination of Special Education Programs," *The Journal of Special Education,* 3 (1969), 376.

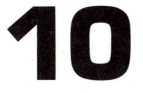

INTERVENTION
An Interaction
Approach

Jim, 25 years old, arrived at the United Cerebral Palsy Association Center with his mother. She hoped that Jim could be provided day services at the center. In the initial conversation with the rehabilitation counselor (intake worker), Jim's mother said that the family had moved to this southern urban city about three months before and really did not yet know the community. After Jim was accepted for services (within three weeks of the initial contact), he was introduced to all the staff members including the therapeutic recreator.

Jim was talkative and had a good sense of humor. However, some of his social skills were poorly developed. He had a limited education, completing the equivalent of the eighth grade. He indicated a strong interest in meeting new friends, developing an intimate relationship, and moving out of his mother's home. After obtaining this initial information, the staff started planning for ways to help Jim look at the reality of his goals and to find ways of obtaining his goals.

INTRODUCTION

Change is a natural function of the human condition. Therapeutic recreators and allied leisure-service personnel are often in the position to help plan, implement, and facilitate change. The *process of intervention* uses various strategies for identifying targets of change, directions in which change is desired, and methods of obtaining desired change.

The process of intervention provides us an excellent opportunity to put into practice the concepts presented in this text. Refer again to the social systems/ecology model discussed in Chapter 1. There it was suggested that therapeutic recreators be aware of the ongoing interaction between people and their environments. The process of intervention, or planned change, is presented within this context.

INTERACTION: THE INDIVIDUAL AND THE ENVIRONMENT

The three major components of the interaction model are the individual, his or her environment, and the interaction between them. The therapeutic recreation professional intervenes in order to facilitate change in the individual and/or the environment. Any intervention strategy is designed with the understanding that there is a direct and reciprocal relationship and subsequent interaction between the individual and the environment. Schulman explains this interaction and relates it to the broad concept of human services. The author states:

> The concept of human services is a philosophy that stresses care for the whole individual and his relation to his environment. It poses a straightforward notion—an individual is influenced by what happens around him; the same individual influences what happens around him. These two kinds of influence make the individual what he is at any one moment.[1]

We recognize that the environment includes many aspects, just as the individual is accepted as a multidimensional being. Auerswald implies that all these dimensions impact upon one another when he suggests that "the symptom, the person, his family and his community interlock."[2] Interlocking relationships are often characterized by various types of support systems, and these systems should not be overlooked by the professional in designing any intervention strategy.

Judith and Michael Lewis have developed a concept called "community counseling"[3] for the delivery of human services. This approach provides support to the interaction model of intervention because its major premise involves the relationship between the individual and the environment. The authors explain this relationship when they discuss the role of community counselors in the process of intervention.

> When helping troubled individuals, community counselors often find themselves working along with their clients to identify the most effective possible sources of support in the natural environment. This must be a joint process, because no one can tell an individual what his or her support system should be. Relationships are only supportive, and only helpful, if people experience them that way. There is no objective truth that can help us to distinguish between a "good" or a "bad" environment. It is the interaction between individuals and their surroundings that is important, and only the people involved can identify the situations in which their own needs are met.[4]

The interaction that takes place between the professional and the individual with a disability requires trust and respect on the part of both parties. The relationship, in order to be most effective, must be based on a belief in the ability of an individual to make self-determined choices. Although the level of this ability varies with each person, the fact that we all possess this ability on some level needs to be acknowledged and included in any intervention strategies.

Intervention is a process that involves a relationship between the professional and the individual with a disability. The Lewises developed two diagrams that depict the intervention process between the counselor and the person being counseled in implementing change within the individual or the environment. These illustrations (see Figs. 10–1 and 10–2) add clarity to the concepts and processes of interaction and intervention.

Both of the processes described by the Lewises stress the importance of support systems and the broad concept of *networking*. We are learning that extending ourselves to others can enhance the intervention process and increase options for the growth and development of individuals with disabilities. In any intervention strategy we must remember the importance of working with individuals with disabilities in an interdependent manner. This means perceiving participants as collaborators in their own growth and development. Lenrow and Burch identify the mutual benefits this interdependent type of relationship can have on the interaction between professionals and participants. The authors state:

> After an initial collaboration, the professional and client are no longer complete strangers to each other. They know what values they have in common and can appeal to in order to keep the working relationship collaborative. So long as there is an expectation that they may work together again after an initial collaboration, they begin to experience themselves as part of an ongoing network, or team, that is committed to certain common values concerning health and well-being. Approaching clients as active participants on a team serves the professionals' utilitarian values: They will get better cooperation, be trusted on a more realistic basis, have more information on which to base effective decisions, and find that clients are more effective in implementing decisions. But such a mode of working with clients also serves nonutilitarian values: health in the positive sense of fulfillment, rather than only the absence of disorder; respect for the resources of all participants; and a sense of community as well as a sense of competence.[5]

The interaction model of intervention consists of six major steps, which are referred to as *process-flow* steps. These steps include the following processes:

1.0 Assess the individual and his or her environment
2.0 Define goals and objectives
3.0 Design plan to modify interaction between disability and environment if necessary

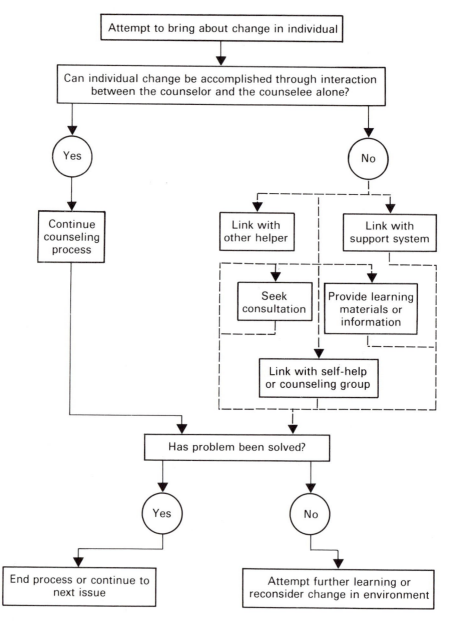

FIGURE 10-1   Facilitating Change Within the Individual. Judith A. Lewis and Michael D. Lewis, *Community Counseling: A Human Service Approach* (New York, N.Y.: John Wiley & Sons, 1977), p. 207.

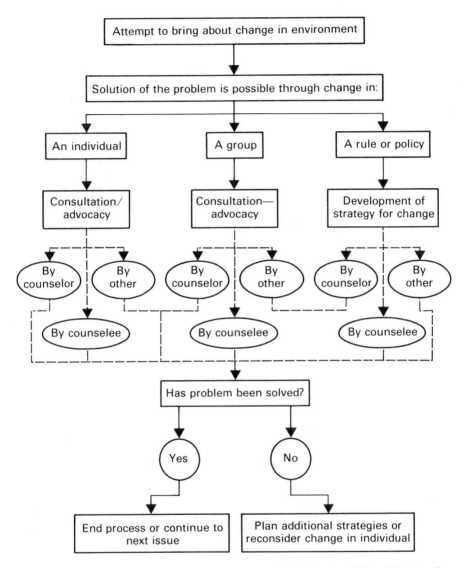

FIGURE 10–2 Facilitating Change Within the Environment. Judith A. Lewis and Michael D. Lewis, *Community Counseling: A Human Service Approach* [New York, N.Y.: John Wiley & Sons, 1977], p. 209.

4.0 Identify and implement intervention strategies and techniques
5.0 Evaluate
6.0 Follow-up of participant

Figure 10–3 illustrates the process-flow steps in the interaction model of intervention.

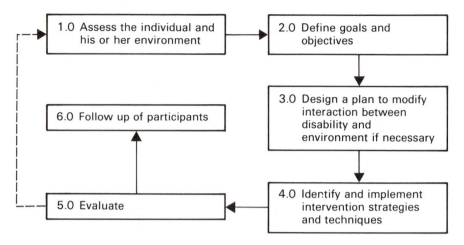

FIGURE 10–3 The Interaction Model of Intervention Process-Flow

The process-flow steps of the model consist of many subprocesses. Each step is broken down into its specific subcomponents and presented below for further clarification.

1.0 Assess the individual and his or her environment.

    1.1 Examine personal assets and liabilities of therapeutic recreator

        Personally assess the following beliefs, leadership values, and interpersonal relationship skills in relation to working with individuals with disabilities:

            level of self-confidence in personal leadership skills

            level of human relations skills (for example, attending, listening, self-disclosure, creativity, openness, compassion, understanding, humor, playfulness, and so forth)

            level and source of professional motivation

            level of belief in the dignity and uniqueness of human beings

            nature of preconceived beliefs about participants and/or their disability

    1.2 Examine ideology of therapeutic recreation delivery system

        Assess the level of existence of the following program philosophies and practices:

            developmental programming

            principles of transfer

            principles of normalization

            task analysis

            integration continuum

            partnerships between disabled and nondisabled people

            role modeling

1.3   Examine ability side of participants/clients
      observe participants' behavior and functional levels
      communicate with participants regarding their needs for support
      assess participants' strengths and weaknesses
      network with allied specialists to gather necessary information about disability and possible intervention strategies

1.4   Examine personal attitudes of participants toward themselves and their disabilities. Design activities to assess and/or communicate with participants regarding their:
      level of intrinsic motivation
      level of independent participation
      level of skill to make self-determined choices
      need for enabling devices
      attitude toward learning
      self-help skills
      cultural and individual lifestyle considerations
      avoidance behaviors
      level of stress

1.5   Assess the environment (physical and social)
Identify factors in the environment that may impact on the individual with a disability:
      architectural barriers
      attitudes of those in client's immediate environment
      social atmosphere of the program environment (degree of respect, open and honest communication, success)
      family and cultural systems
      school, community, and organizational systems
      adaptive equipment and devices
      support services

1.6   Identify environmental demands, expectations on participants (consider ability assessment data in steps 1.3, 1.4, 1.5)
      variation in the human condition and impact of environment
      functional and behavioral requirements for activity and independence in environment
      inadequacies or behavioral deficits in relation to the environment
      negative, environmentally related consequences of the ability

1.7   Determine available resources
      network with other community groups/agencies, specialists, and generalists
      identify instructional materials
      identify parent groups and organizations
      identify self-help, advocacy groups

2.0   Define goals and objectives.
      identify mutually acceptable ends
      individualize goals and objectives
      communicate and clarify goals and objectives with participant

3.0   Design plan to modify interaction between disability and environment if necessary.

> eliminate or modify environmental barriers (social/physical)
>
> reassess personal attitudes of staff and participants

4.0   Identify and implement intervention strategies and techniques. (Use strategies that incorporate the following practices and ideologies):

> developmental learning
>
> transfer principles
>
> intrinsic motivation
>
> social stimulation in environments
>
> human relations
>
> cooperative participation
>
> explanation/examples
>
> open and honest communication
>
> activity analysis and modification
>
> challenge and risk taking
>
> creative problem solving
>
> independent participation
>
> responsible social behavior
>
> environmental barrier removal
>
> leisure education and counseling

5.0   Evaluate.

> formative
>
> summative
>
> evaluate individual progress
>
> evaluate the services provided

6.0   Follow-up of participant.

> assist participant in making transition to home-based, leisure-oriented environment
>
> evaluate transferability of individual's program to home environment
>
> assist in connecting individual to available resources

This review of the process-flow steps is intended to assist the reader in gaining a picture of the entire *process* of intervention. The next section highlights some of the important issues and techniques involved in intervention. It will also refer to Jim, who was introduced at the beginning of the chapter, to illustrate how the process works.

ASSESSMENT

Assessment of the Individual

Assessment refers to that part of the process whereby data are collected regarding the individual. A variety of sources are tapped to generate information that is useful, relevant, and accurate. Medical records, written histories, and comments made by both family members and others who know the person serve as primary sources. Of course, the client will provide the most significant information, either through direct conversation or interviewing, observation of the individual in a variety of situations, and by paper and pencil or other forms of testing.

What we must remember about assessment is that the professional/ practitioner is prone to possessing a biased frame of reference. We may expect, for example, that individuals will experience certain types of "problems" based upon the fact that they are seeking treatment in a specific setting. The way we interpret behaviors or skills may also reflect the nature of the environment in which we work.

As an example of the issue raised here, Rosenhan published what is now a classic study, in which he tried to determine whether the sane could be distinguished from the insane by professionals in psychiatric hospitals. He selected eight sane people and instructed them to seek admission into mental health hospitals. The subjects who secretly gained admission into these settings falsified their names and occupations. Each complained to admissions personnel that they heard "empty" and "hollow" voices. This was the extent of their "symptoms."

The results: admittance to psychiatric hospitals and *diagnosis* as *schizophrenic*. The subjects were instructed to behave normally if they were admitted. Regardless of their "good behavior," it took on the average 19 days for them to be released, with the label "schizophrenia in remission." It was additionally reported that actual patients detected the fake patients ("you're not crazy"), yet staff viewed the open note-taking by subjects as a symptom of abnormality.[6]

Another example of how our perspectives tend to change as a result of the environment involves sexual contact. If one is in a hospital bed with the door closed, is sexual contact appropriate? Would a man found caressing his wife who came to visit him in the hospital be considered deviant or a troublemaker by the hospital staff? In other words, behaviors that are acceptable in daily life and practiced by nonstigmatized people may not be perceived as appropriate in medical, institutional, or other settings.

Another consideration in observing behaviors as part of assessment is that individuals tend to act or react differently in unfamiliar settings. Anxiety, fear, confusion, isolation, and other very real human experiences are likely to be manifest in behaviors that are not part of an individual's usual repertoire of behavior. "Behavioral responsiveness to settings is selected for because appropriateness of behavior is crucial to adaptation in many settings."[7] In other words, behavior is largely dependent upon the setting in which it occurs. Changing the environment may change the behavior; therefore, it is not defensible to assess a person's performance—period. Rather, we have to assess performance by setting because variations in settings produce variations in performance![8]

What is assessed in the area of therapeutic recreation? This introductory text cannot cover this question comprehensively, but new developments in the field are particularly worthy of attention here.

Traditionally, assessment has focused on eliciting individual interests in specific activities, and identifying present and desired skill levels needed for certain leisure activities; deciphering how a person spends his or her "free time"; attempting to determine why a person engages in certain kinds of activities, be they socially acceptable or not; and observing social-interaction behaviors. We have also often borrowed from allied fields, particularly occupational therapy and special education, to determine motor skills; developmental behaviors, such as cognitive and language development; self-help skills (for example, feeding, toileting, personal hygiene) and related behaviors. Of course, it is unnecessary to duplicate assessments implemented by other professionals if the results are accessible.

In a valuable contribution to the field, Peter Witt and Gary Ellis, both leaders and forward thinkers in the leisure sciences, tackled the problem of assessment. Utilizing the most recent literature and research, they systematically attempted to identify those underlying human dimensions that contributed to or restricted the leisure experience. By adopting the "leisure as a state of mind" concept, they identified and put into operation those conditions that they suggest comprise "leisure functioning." These components were translated into scales in the Leisure Diagnostic Battery and are listed along with a brief description of each in Table 10-1.

This diagnostic battery provides us with the first solid, conceptually developed, and widely tested assessment tool in the field.

Assessment of the Environment

In addition to adequate knowledge about the client, information on the individual's living environment is also essential to understanding the factors that regularly impact upon that person. For example, an adolescent male living in a rural convalescent home confronts different realities from that of an adolescent male living with his natural family in a suburban setting. To be viable, any individual program plan (IPP) must take into account the context in which individuals find themselves.

Another reason for gathering data on an individual's environment is that barriers may exist within that environment which will interfere substantially with a person's independence. While therapeutic recreators are not in a position to tackle all environmental problems, they may be able to address some problem areas, such as a lack of leisure resources within the home environment.

Data about home/work/school/community environments can be obtained through many of the same sources that provide information on the individual. The therapeutic recreator may find it necessary to make on-site visits to significant settings of the clients. This assessment is important be-

TABLE 10-1 The Leisure Diagnostic Battery

SECTION 1: PRELIMINARY ASSESSMENT INSTRUMENTS TO DETERMINE "DOES A PROBLEM EXIST?"

SCALE	DESCRIPTION/PURPOSE
A. Perceived Leisure Competence	To determine the individual's perception of his or her own level of physical, social, cognitive, and general competence in leisure experiences.
B. Voluntary-Reward Motivation for Involvement in Leisure Experiences	To determine the degree to which individuals are internally motivated to undertake leisure activities and experiences vs. the degree to which they are influenced by extrinsic rewards.
C. Perceived Leisure Control	To determine whether individuals believe that their leisure is primarily under their own control or is under the control of events, persons, or circumstances beyond themselves.
D. Leisure Needs	To determine the ability an individual has to meet fundamental needs via leisure experiences.
E. Depth of Involvement in Leisure	To determine the degree of involvement an individual is able to achieve during leisure experiences.
F. Playfulness	To determine the degree to which an individual may be considered playful, i.e., spontaneous (social, physical, cognitive), and showing a sense of humor and manifest joy.
G. Barriers to Leisure Experiences	To determine problems that an individual encounters when trying to select or participate in leisure experiences.
H. Leisure Preferences	To determine the individual's patterns of selection among activities within five domains (outdoor/nature; music/dance/drama; sports; arts/crafts/hobbies; and mental/linguistic). In addition, this scale measures preference for mode or style of involvement in three cases (individual-group; risk/nonrisk; and active-passive).
I. Knowledge of Leisure	To determine the individual's knowledge of specific information concerning leisure opportunities. This information includes information related to leisure opportunities, the cost, who can participate, where, when, and what.

Gary Ellis and Peter Witt, *The Leisure Diagnostic Battery Users Guide* (Denton, Tex.: Division of Recreation and Leisure Studies, North Texas State University, August 1982), pp. 4–5.

cause we expect the benefits of the services we provide to extend beyond the boundaries of the program itself. This aspect of the assessment, then, provides a context for implementing the entire IPP.

The Program Analysis of Service Systems (PASS) is an assessment instrument, based upon the principles of normalization, designed to assess the environment.[9] It has been adapted for use in leisure service programs. The Assessment of Environmental Barriers to Leisure Experiences (AEBLE), developed at North Texas University in conjunction with the Leisure Diagnostic Battery, focuses on how the individual consumer perceives his or her environment.[10] To date, few such tools exist in leisure services.

It is the belief of the authors that both the facility/program environment and the immediate personal environment of each individual in service settings should be considered as integral to the individual plan devised by therapeutic recreation staff. Although the process used in developing an "environmental action plan" is still in its infancy, the steps of intervention—environmentally focused assessment goals (which support the individual); design of the action plan, (what, where, when, who); implementation of the plan; evaluation and follow-up—can each be applied to the environment.

Regardless of the focus of the assessment, the client/patient/consumer should be involved to the maximum extent possible. The more he/she is able to take responsibility in generating data, the more likely that person is to have a sense of ownership and desire to participate in the change process.

The information in Table 10–2 indicates the information the therapeutic recreator might obtain during the assessment phase.

Synthesis of Assessment

Jim is verbal, often dominating the conversation, and uses language and jokes that are offensive to observers. He has always lived with his mother

TABLE 10–2 Assessment

FOCUS: JIM	FOCUS: JIM'S ENVIRONMENT
MAIN SOURCES OF INFORMATION:	MAIN SOURCES OF INFORMATION:
Jim his mother his brother historical/medical records assessments of allied health personnel	Jim his mother his brother allied health personnel
TECHNIQUES, TOOLS OF ASSESSMENT	TECHNIQUES, TOOLS OF ASSESSMENT
LDB and AEBLE Instruments Observation of Jim interacting with peers, staff, family Interviews	Observing of family members interacting with Jim Visitation to home Interviews

and younger brother. The family has recently moved to a large urban area from a small rural area in order to be close to extended family members. Jim's father died approximately eight months before the move.

Jim attended a special-education program. He lacks basic writing and mathematical skills. He uses a wheelchair.

Jim expresses an interest to live on his own or with another person in his own apartment. He has not worked and is unclear about job interests. However, he does like to do things with his hands and he especially enjoys cooking.

Jim also expresses an interest in having a romantic relationship, but he has never had an unsupervised social-sexual relationship.

His mother states that she is concerned about Jim's being more independent, and she is fearful he will be taken advantage of or otherwise hurt. She says that he will never be able to work or live independently. She expresses interest in having the staff help Jim be more realistic about his goals.

IDENTIFICATION OF GOALS AND OBJECTIVES

Based upon the analysis of the information generated, goals and objectives identify short- and long-term ends for which the client will strive. In therapeutic recreation, these can be as diverse as the development of skills enabling a person to successfully participate in a card game with three other people, to learning particular activity skills (photography, canoeing, badminton, yoga) to learning how to block out extraneous sounds in order to be attentive in a game situation. Other goals may relate to increasing one's ability to relax, to get to and from a park independently, to increase one's reliability as a volunteer, to develop a sense of affiliation with a group, or to increase one's sense of competence in a social setting.

Objectives are yet more specific statements of expected outcomes, derived specifically from the goals. Practitioners in the health and helping professions have been urged to state objectives in behavioral terms, that is, in terms of specific behaviors. Objectives are to be demonstrated within a specified period of time and under a described set of conditions. The behavioral approach has a number of benefits, including observable results, which are useful in documenting progress (related to accountability). A major limitation of this approach is engendered by the very nature of leisure, particularly the "state of mind" concept and the nature of the play experience. How does a person who is developing "perceived competence" act? Given the complexity and internal nature of the leisure phenomenon, developing other approaches to selecting and identifying individually desired outcomes is a continuing challenge within therapeutic recreation.

Once again, the importance of the patient/client's assuming an active role in establishing goals and objectives cannot be overestimated.

Table 10–3 reveals possible goals and objectives toward which Jim could

TABLE 10–3 Goals and Objectives of Individual Program Plan

FOCUS: JIM	FOCUS: JIM'S ENVIRONMENT
GOAL:	GOAL:
Increase Jim's social competence	Increase opportunities for Jim to go into community without his mother.
OBJECTIVE	OBJECTIVE
At the end of three weeks, Jim will demonstrate the ability to interact appropriately with verbal peers at the center. Specifically, he will: a. Maintain a two-way conversation on a topic of mutual interest for at least eight minutes when asked by the therapeutic recreator. b. Refrain from telling offensive jokes, as determined by those with whom he is interacting.	At the end of four weeks, Jim's mother will give permission for Jim to attend a community-based event with a person in his age bracket.

work. You will note that the goals and objectives are based on the information generated through the assessment.

THE DESIGN OF THE PLAN

Focus: the individual. The next step in individualizing program plans is to select activities or modalities that will assist the individual in attaining his or her goals and objectives: selecting the manner in which these modalities will be implemented (frequency, length of time, facilitation method used, and site where activity will take place). The design serves to provide continuity to the implementation of the treatment and serves as a vehicle for communication. Moreover, the design takes into account personal, cultural, and other lifestyle considerations, such as age, ethnicity, religious beliefs, educational level, socioeconomic status, the preferred lifestyle, and the values of the community in which the individual resides.

Focus: the physical environment. Elements of physical design, esthetics, textures, fragrances, and safety are among the environmental characteristics considered crucial in environments, particularly those concerned with learning and play.

Often we find ourselves using physical environments that are not particularly desirable for our uses. Rooms may be too small; long, narrow hallways and cemented yards are examples of physical characteristics that service providers may have to contend with. Consequently, personal creativity is an important asset under these conditions, for our task is to make the environment as comfortable, usable, and positive as possible. Clients/consumers should also have opportunities for creating an environment that is satisfying. For example, in long-term settings, such as day programs for adults with chronic mental illness, the clients can help plan, design, and conceive an environment that facilitates social interaction, provides unobstructed room for diverse activities, and protects personal privacy. Using guided imagery, we can help clients identify those environments in which they feel good. From them, we can elicit colors and shapes, seating arrangements, functional items, such as bookshelves or tables, and a host of other characteristics that will help create an enabling environment. Through the use of models and maps (which clients can help to create), we can help to arrange rooms to be more functional in meeting both personal and program needs.

In short-term environments, where there is a relatively rapid turnover of participants (for example, programs for individuals who are dealing with alcoholism or other forms of chemical dependence), even minor environmental changes, such as the use of personal pictures, can help personalize space. By personalizing our living, working, and playing space, we gain some amount of personal control and identity.

Modified environments should be based on individual program plans: What type of an environment will assist the individual in interacting with peers? In being more mobile? In concentrating on the development of certain skills? The therapeutic recreation specialist can establish, even within the strict confines dictated by the administration, a physical environment that provides users with positive mental images and enhances a harmonious relationship between the participant and the world.

Again, one needs to look beyond the program space itself. Parents, managers of group homes, and other residential-care personnel may welcome suggestions for modifying the home environment to promote positive play and leisure behavior.

Focus: the social environment.   Because the social environment is composed of a complex array of verbal and nonverbal interpersonal interactions, professionals can establish a social environment that is nurturing and supportive by virtue of their own behaviors and communication and by the way in which they guide the behaviors and expressions of other program participants.

The social environment created by the home, be it a natural or foster family, or by an institutional environment is crucial to the long-term development and growth of the person. Although therapeutic recreation specialists may not be equipped to deal effectively with hostile home environments, they can be alert to such situations and work with allied professionals, such

TABLE 10–4   Design of Program Plan

FOCUS: JIM	FOCUS: JIM'S ENVIRONMENT
1. Jim will initially discuss appropriate social interaction behaviors with therapeutic recreator for 30 minutes.	1. The therapeutic recreator and rehabilitation counselor will request visit to Jim's home.
2. Jim will participate in the "Friends" groups twice a week. Within this structured social group, Jim will be given verbal cues regarding appropriate social interaction. Appropriate behavior (maintaining eye contact, using nonsexual words, listening behavior, taking turns speaking) will be encouraged by the therapeutic recreator.	2. Both the therapeutic recreator and rehabilitation counselor will talk to Jim's mother about her perceptions of Jim and suggest that he has potential for more independence.
3. The therapeutic recreator will also observe Jim informally (during lunch, unstructured times).	3. Meetings with mother will be scheduled regularly, as needed, to provide her support and information.
4. Jim will meet weekly with the therapeutic recreator to receive feedback and discuss his own perceptions of his behavior. Role-playing will be used during these one-on-one sessions.	4. The therapeutic recreator will contact a member of the Young Adults group (self-help group of disabled adults who are working toward independence) to invite Jim to a meeting and community outing.
	5. Mother will be invited to a center program to observe Jim's behavior and his self-help skills.

as social workers, in assisting families to create more healthful and playful atmospheres. Certainly the efforts of a team will likely be most effective in working in any familial environment.

Table 10–4 continues the program plan for Jim. Again, the activities and modalities selected should follow naturally from the goals and objectives.

IMPLEMENTATION

The design of the plan is implemented according to the details outlined. The therapeutic recreator should be extremely observant during the implementation process as new data may be generated that require an adjustment in the plan; and feedback data can be obtained to help determine the efficiency, adequacy, and helpfulness of the design. In both therapeutic recreation and leisure service settings, the outcome of the activity or experience (whether the game is won or lost; whether the music was sung on key) is not the issue. Rather, *what happened to the individual* is the crux of the service; feelings, social behaviors, gains in perceived competence, perceived control, and intrinsic motivation are the focus of programs. Recreation is uniquely suitable for increasing a sense of control, particularly under conditions that are controlled by others—as in an institutional setting. Often, a "debriefing" between the therapeutic recreator and client will occur after the treatment sessions to discuss what happened "below the surface" of the experience.

EVALUATION AND FEEDBACK

Evaluation (for the purposes of this discussion) refers to the gathering of data about progress of the individual toward maximum leisure functioning, so that decisions about the details of service delivery can be made. Evaluation occurs within every component of the individualization process. The feedback of data from this kind of evaluation (called *formative evaluation*) allows the practitioner to make necessary adjustments in the program plan while it is being designed and implemented. *Summative evaluation* occurs at the end of a treatment plan (or at the termination of a preselected time period) and makes it possible to determine whether the individual's goals and objectives have been realized. If actual progress exceeds or falls short of anticipated outcomes, the plan can be redesigned for the next program cycle, as appropriate.

Evaluating individual progress is conducted by determining the extent to which a person has reached his or her objectives. Each objective, then, provides the criteria by which progress is determined and through which the effectiveness of service delivery is documented.

Evaluation of individual progress is an essential element of the change process. Yet it is often done informally, if at all. As practitioners become cognizant of the inherent nature of evaluation in individualizing programs, it will become a more natural element in practice, designed directly into the program plan.

Table 10–5 provides an example of information gathered through the

TABLE 10–5 Evaluation of Client Progress

FOCUS: JIM	FOCUS: JIM'S ENVIRONMENT
1. At the end of three weeks, Jim achieved the objectives and has maintained appropriate social behavior as defined by the objectives.	1. Jim's mother reluctantly gave permission for Jim to attend a community-based event. She put several restrictions on the outings, including a 10 P.M. curfew, and no alcoholic beverages. After three events, covering a period of six weeks, she gave him a 10:30 curfew.
2. The next step should focus on: a. Jim's social skills during unstructured times. b. Jim's social skills with peers outside of the center.	2. Jim's mother expressed considerable anger at the center staff for encouraging his social activity. This, in turn, has caused some tension for Jim at home. Recommend a meeting with Jim and his mother to discuss this issue.

evaluation. In most treatment settings, progress is documented in individual charts and much more specific information is included.

FOLLOW-UP

The process of *follow-up* recognizes the importance of "following through" with an individual making a transition from one environment to another. It is a logical step in individualized services because persons receiving treatment sometimes fall into the inevitable gap between services, which can result in personal regression, social isolation, and debilitative conditions.

Change-oriented individualized programs are intended to result in benefits that supersede the boundaries of the program itself. Individuals tend to participate in residential or outpatient rehabilitative services for a relatively short period of time. What faces the postrehabilitation individual is a lifetime of maximizing abilities and minimizing limitations within school, work, play, home, and various other environments. For service providers to be successful in helping clients "live life to its maximum," providers can assist the individual in making useful connections with specialized and generic services, with self-help groups, and in experiencing other meaningful opportunities. The transition from one setting to another can be either a debilitating or a growth-oriented experience, depending upon the manner in which it is handled. Therapeutic recreation personnel can be effective in assisting in the follow-up process by being aware of resources that exist in the individual's community (see Table 10–6).

INDIVIDUALIZING: THE WRITTEN PLAN

Throughout this discussion, we have emphasized working with the *individual* consumer in designing and implementing intervention strategies. At the heart of the personal change process that has meaning for the consumer is the art and science of *individualizing* goals, services, and strategies. Effective intervention requires that the service provider focus on the abilities, interests,

TABLE 10–6 Follow-Up

FOCUS: JIM	FOCUS: JIM'S ENVIRONMENT
1. Talk with Jim about his new experiences.	1. Keep open lines of communication with his mother.
2. Define new objectives.	2. Contact member of Young Adults group for feedback and suggestions.

lifestyle, concerns, aspirations, and problems of the individual consumer; on the characteristics of the environment; and on the selection of strategies that will likely result in positive change. Herein lies one of the major challenges confronting practitioners.

Beyond this challenge is the demand for accountability for our actions. Individualization has resulted largely because we must be able to document the effects of our services. By individualizing, we are more likely to be able to identify specific needs, define desirable goals and objectives, select and implement appropriate techniques directed toward the attainment of those objectives, and observe the resulting degree of success. In some settings, individualized plans are required in order to meet legislative mandates and to qualify for funding. The terms applied to these plans of action differ slightly according to the settings in which services are delivered and according to their primary objectives. The following list sets forth terms and their contexts.

Term	Where Used
Individualized Education Plan (IEP)	Schools
Individualized Treatment Plan (ITP)	Clinical/Rehabilitation settings/ Hospitals
Individualized Service Plan (ISP)/	Residential centers
Individualized Program Plan (IPP)	Group homes
	Day centers

Typically, these plans are designed in a similar manner, utilizing comprehensive information on the client/consumer/patient as a prerequisite to developing a plan of action to realize particular individual goals. The plan, then, is a blueprint for specifying the details—the where, when, who, what of service delivery. To be most effective, a program plan is reevaluated on a regular basis to ensure that the services continue to meet the individual's needs.

In a comprehensive plan, the services of different disciplines will be incorporated, including those of therapeutic recreation. In other cases, therapeutic recreation will have a separate IPP. The written document in the form of a program plan is a visible manifestation of the intervention process. In many settings, once an individual has been assessed and has goals and objectives, he or she will participate in already existing small-group therapeutic recreation programs with other individuals having similar objectives.

SUMMARY

This chapter discussed the process of intervention from an interaction perspective. The reader is cautioned to recognize the interaction between individuals and their environments and to focus on strategies for change within this context. Six major steps, along with various substeps, were cited as comprising the change/intervention process, regardless of the target of change. Several considerations in intervention were highlighted.

The process of designing intervention plans is both an art and a science. Great strides have been made in the profession over the last decade to refine the tools and strategies for designing effective interventions.

DISCUSSION QUESTIONS

10-1. What is meant by "the process of intervention"?

10-2. What would you expect to take place in the relationship between the consumer/client and the therapeutic recreation specialist during the intervention process?

10-3. What is the purpose of the following major steps of the intervention process?
assessment
identification of goals and objectives
design of the plan
implementation of the plan
evaluation
follow-up of the individual

10-4. How does this process apply to:
a. the individual?
b. the individual's environment?

CASE STUDY

Work in teams of two. Decide which person will initially role-play the therapeutic recreator, and which will role-play the consumer/client. You will also reverse roles so that each person plays both roles. As a "team" you will undertake the intervention process on behalf of the client. The client should identify some real-life issue that he or she would like to address related to leisure and well-being. For example, perhaps the client would like to do the following: engage in some pleasurable form of physical activity on a regular basis; learn a new leisure skill; find a way to take some time for personal reflection on a daily basis. Once the target area is identified, the therapeutic recreator should begin the intervention process.

Steps 1 to 4 below probably can occur in one stage. Step 4 may take from one to two weeks, depending upon the nature of your plan. The final steps (5 and 6) can take place in one stage.

a. Start with an informal assessment. What kinds of questions might you want to ask that would be helpful in developing a plan of action? Develop a list of questions or use another form of assessment that is appropriate. The therapeutic recreator and client will work closely together throughout this activity. Write down the data that are gathered. Discuss what the data mean. This will require that you do some interpretation of the data. Be sure to check it out with the client.

b. Identify one goal that reflects the data that you gathered. Then, develop one or two specific objectives from the goal. The objectives will be the basis of the evaluation, so make certain that you can measure whether or not the objectives have been attained.

c. Design a plan for the client to implement. This plan should be designed to help that individual meet his or her objective within a reasonable amount of time. For purposes of this activity, the plan could take one to two weeks.

d. The client implements the program within the specified amount of time. Check-in points with the therapeutic recreator during the implementation stage will assist both team members in monitoring progress.

e. The therapeutic recreator and client together evaluate the effectiveness of the plan. Did the client attain his or her objective? Why or why not?

f. How would you follow up with this particular client?

Note:

1. The team members can reverse roles after the first team has done steps *a* to *c*. That will allow both individuals to implement their plan during the same one- to two-week time frame. Of course, this means that both individuals will play two roles simultaneously.

2. This activity does not stress the technical skills necessary in developing a clinical intervention process. Rather, the emphasis is on understanding the overall process. Therefore, students are encouraged to discuss the experience with the instructor, noting areas of difficulty.

3. What does it feel like to be the "helper" in this process? What does it feel like to be the "client"?

NOTES

[1]E. D. Shulman, *Intervention in the Human Services* (St. Louis: The C.B. Mosby Company, 1974), p. 4.

[2]E. H. Auerswald, "Interdisciplinary versus Ecological Approach," *Family Process,* 7, No. 2 (1967), 207.

[3]Judith A. Lewis and Michael D. Lewis, *Community Counseling: A Human Service Approach,* 2nd ed. (New York: John Wiley & Sons, 1983).

[4]Ibid, p. 201.

[5]Peter B. Lenrow and Rosemary W. Burch, "Mutual Aid and Professional Services: Opposing or Complementary?", in *Social Networks and Social Support,* ed. Benjamin H. Gottlieb (Beverly Hills, Calif.: Sage Publications, 1981), pp. 252-253.

[6]Seppo E. Iso-Ahola, *The Social-Psychology of Leisure and Recreation* (Dubuque, Iowa: Wm. C. Brown, 1980).

[7]Edwin P. Willems, "Behavioral Ecology and Health Status and Care," in *Human Behavior and Environment: Advances in Theory and Research*, eds. Irwin Altman and Joachim Wohlwill (New York: Plenum Press, 1976), p. 239.

[8]Ibid., p. 242.

[9]W. Wolfensberger and L. Glenn, *Program Analysis of Service Systems (PASS): A Method for the Quantitative Evaluation of Human Services*, 3rd ed. (Toronto: National Institute on Mental Retardation, 1978).

[10]Peter Witt and David Compton, "Assessment of Environmental Barriers to Leisure Experiences" (Denton, Tex.: North Texas State University, Division of Recreation and Leisure Studies, 1982).

11

THERAPEUTIC RECREATION IN REHABILITATION

Franklin was driving home late one night after work. He fell asleep at the wheel and rammed his car into a bridge. He survived with severe trauma to the brain. At 25 years of age, he will spend the next couple of weeks in acute care, followed by several months in rehabilitation. He has lost the typical brain functions of memory, judgment, and visual-social perception. He and the rehabilitation team will work to assess what strengths and capabilities remain intact and what functions can be redeveloped.

Judith, a 43-year-old administrator for a small company, was diagnosed with lung cancer eight months ago. She recently resigned from her position and is receiving chemotherapy treatment on an outpatient basis at the community hospital. Her spirits are sagging; she is losing some hair and she often feels "lousy." Her prognosis is not favorable, and her disease continues to grow. She's concerned about her two teenage children, who are very upset and confused about her illness. "When the time comes," says Judith, "I want to die at home, if possible. But I don't know if the kids can handle it."

Amy is in her eighties. Until she fell and broke a hip and arm, she lived independently. Neighbors in her apartment complex looked in on her regularly. She has just been placed in an intermediate care facility. Although dismayed that she had to leave her home, she is optimistic about healing quickly and returning to her typical life pattern. In the meantime, her neighbors occasionally visit. She's indicated that she is a bit bored and has a "nagging feeling" that maybe she'll never again be fully independent.

What are the roles of therapeutic recreators in these situations? How can these individuals be helped? What kind of factors should be taken into consideration when planning services? How can therapeutic recreators be effective?

INTRODUCTION

This chapter will emphasize the nature of rehabilitative/habilitative intervention in recreation and the use of basic strategies that can be effective in reaching rehabilitative goals. While the reader may be inclined to think of rehabilitation in terms of setting alone (hospital, rehabilitation center, and so forth), this process is not restricted to any specific environment. Rehabilitation, as a function, can occur in clinical, educational, home, or other settings.

What is stressed in this chapter is the *total* context of rehabilitation: the patient/client; the models of service delivery; the practices; the issues; the physical, emotional, and social environment; and the service providers. Recall the importance of acknowledging the broader picture and the interaction of the various elements in the rehabilitation system as we provide a picture of the contribution of therapeutic recreation services.

THE FUNCTION OF REHABILITATION/HABILITATION

Rehabilitation is a dynamic process with the purpose of *restoring an individual to maximum physical, mental, emotional functioning and to a valued status and role in society.*[1] This process is typically initiated after a catastrophic disease or traumatic accident that has left a previously able-bodied person with new life conditions, such as spinal cord injury, head injury, or amputation. *Habilitation* refers to the above process when it is directed toward a person who is congenitally disabled or disabled in the early developmental years. (For purposes of brevity, the term *rehabilitation* will be used throughout the chapter.) From a holistic perspective of the individual, rehabilitation encompasses: (1) physical rehabilitation (medication, surgery, exercises, prostheses, and survival technology, such as dialysis machines); (2) vocational rehabilitation (work adjustment, job placement); (3) social rehabilitation (social-skill development, sex therapy, activities of daily living, leisure development); and (4) psychological rehabilitation (counseling, psychotherapy, emotional support).[2] As an individual-oriented process, it addresses the whole person by recognizing that disability can affect every aspect of life.

TWO DIVERGENT HEALTH SERVICE MODELS: THERAPY AND HOLISTIC HEALING

Therapeutic recreation services are put into practice inside larger agencies, organizations, or institutions that are based on what Gerald O'Morrow calls "human service models." He suggests that human service models "differ in historical development, in orientation, in their mode of intervention and in the professional groups that dominate."[3] Further, it can be said that they differ in values. A multitude of such models exist, though they tend not to be mutually exclusive. This section will examine two such models.

Therapy/Medical Model

This traditional model is dominated by the medical profession, which stresses the use of medicine and surgical procedures to defeat illness and correct individual deficiencies. At the core of this approach is the doctor who prescribes all care; other health professionals act in supportive roles and deliver services only as directed. The patient typically assumes a passive profile while the attending professionals provide care and, when possible, cure. Physical therapy, occupational therapy, and speech therapy are examples of allied health professions that have evolved according to this model. Politically, economically, and legally, the therapy/medical model has been a powerful and dominant model of health care service in the United States.

In a strict medical environment, the actions of the therapeutic recreator are restricted to doctor's orders. In some instances, where the doctor is aware of the contribution of recreation and the role of leisure in life, recreation therapy will play an important rehabilitation function. In situations where the doctor is not aware of its benefits, therapeutic recreation may not be a part of the treatment. Obviously the ability of therapeutic recreators to articulate the value of leisure to allied health and medical professions is extremely important.

The way in which recreation functions in a rehabilitation model varies. According to Gunn and Peterson, the goal of recreation therapy/rehabilitation is "to improve the functional ability" or the "improvement of a client's physical, social, mental and/or emotional behaviors"[4] as an antecedent to satisfactory leisure behavior. Recreation is used as a tool to attain desirable goals. It is an integral component of the entire rehabilitation process, as prescribed by the primary physician. The following case study exemplifies this perspective.

Jon, age 10, has recently entered a residential, treatment-oriented hospital school, where he will reside for approximately 10 weeks. As a result of cerebral palsy, he has little functional use of his legs. His doctors believe that with a series of surgical procedures, he will be able to ambulate with the use of crutches. Jon has average intelligence and attends fifth grade. He displays immature social skills, rarely interacting positively with peers. After a thorough assessment with input from various health care staff, recreation therapy is prescribed, with the major goal of improving Jon's social interaction skills. After surgery, recreation therapy will also be prescribed to support mobility skills being developed by the physical therapist.

The recreation therapist initially works with Jon individually for 20 minutes after school three times a week. They talk about Jon's interests, his friends, and his activities over table games. Twice a week, the recreation therapist (R.T.) asks Jon to invite his roommate or another child to play cards or to do other activities with them. The R.T. gives verbal feedback to both children and helps them find ways to do things together successfully.

The R.T. anticipates that in two to three weeks, he will encourage Jon to join in small-group activities and outings. He is careful to record Jon's behavior in social settings and to find strategies that will help the young patient learn to make and keep friends.

In some rehabilitation facilities, "recreation" is considered a peripheral "luxury" rather than an integral treatment component. In these situations, the specialist may provide primarily diversionary activities to keep patients from being bored and to give treatment staff time away from the patients. Recreation comes after the "important" work of the day and on weekends. Activities are often done in medium to large groups with no specific treatment goals in mind. Staff is sometimes referred to as "activity people" or "play ladies." This custodial-oriented approach offers little to the consumer and should not be confused with a treatment-oriented modality.

On the other hand, patients in rehabilitation settings also need relaxation, freedom to choose, and opportunities for non-goal-oriented experiences. These opportunities may well occur during evening and weekend hours.

The National Therapeutic Recreation Society and several state professional organizations have been active in setting guidelines and standards for the provision of recreation therapy services within rehabilitation settings. Members of the organization have worked closely with other agencies, such as the Joint Council on Accreditation of Hospitals, to ensure that quality services are provided by qualified personnel. These activities, along with the committed work of many professionals, have helped to raise the awareness of allied health personnel of the value of quality services and to develop higher levels of services.

The Holistic Healing Model

The *holistic healing model* offers a profound contrast to traditional health services. While the concept can be traced back to Hippocrates, who believed each person needed to be understood as a whole, the contemporary interpretation has blossomed from the consumer movement of the late 1960s. Today, it denotes an approach to understanding the whole person in his or her environment and the use of a variety of healing and health-promoting practices.[5] Here, health refers to that global concept engendered by the term "quality of life." Holistic healing means

> . . . treating the whole person, helping the person to bring mental/emotional, physical, social and spiritual dimensions of his or her being into greater harmony . . . in as much as possible, placing reliance on treatment modalities that foster the self-regenerative and self-reparatory processes of natural healing.[6]

Several basic principles of holistic healing have been set forth by Otto and Knight, pioneers in the movement. The eight principles enumerated below are a synthesis of their ideas:[7]

1. Recognition that every human being has vast untapped potentials, resources, and powers is inherent in holistic healing.

It is widely accepted that we use only a fraction (some suggest less than 10 percent) of our human capacities. While we gain knowledge daily about our existence, human beings are essentially "mysteries." However, by drawing from the systems perspective described in Chapter 1, we can begin to view each individual as a complex configuration of interacting components. As a component of larger social systems, we interact in a multitude of ways with other complex human beings. From this perspective, Otto and Knight suggest that "individual human energy systems can also become conduits of therapeutic power and healing."[8]

2. The fostering of self-awareness and self-understanding can play a vital role in the healing process.

The human potential movement has fostered thousands of books, periodicals, workshops, and self-help organizations aimed at promoting self-understanding. Those activities which are authentic are based upon the premise that the more we understand our internal mechanisms and responses to the environment, the greater power we have in healing ourselves—physically, mentally, socially, spiritually, and emotionally.

3. Placing reliance on the capacities and resources of the person seeking health is a key factor in mobilizing the healing process.

The health team serves primarily as a facilitator, enabling the individual to identify, develop, and tap personal resources for the purposes of health. The individual is perceived as a goal-seeking being who possesses internal resources that can serve to promote self-healing.

4. The interpersonal relationship environment is an integral part of the treatment program and is of outstanding importance throughout the process of healing.

The physical and social environment plays a crucial role in furnishing a nurturing and supportive emotional environment. The warmth, empathy, and understanding provided by healing personnel and members of the individual's social or family network can lead to optimal recovery.

5. Maximal use needs to be made of self-regulating processes and therapies within the dynamics of a disease process before that process reaches the point where major chemotherapy or surgical treatment is required.

Self-regulatory processes, such as relaxation, biofeedback training, and health-producing foods, can accelerate an individual's recovery by activating the person's natural healing processes.

6. Holistic healing makes optimal use of the dynamics and therapeutic forces inherent in group interaction and group work.

A well-facilitated group can serve as a potent vehicle for healing by furnishing a supportive emotional climate, providing reinforcement for learning new behaviors and limiting disease-producing behaviors, and providing a structure through which friendships can be formed. In an era in which people's isolation has become a serious social concern, groups can help individuals reduce estrangement from themselves and from one another by encouraging connections.

7. Recognizing the integrative aspect of life, holistic healing also addresses itself to the quality of a person's life by fostering exploration of the personal lifestyle, to bring values, goals, aspirations, and personal functioning into increased harmony.

Conflict and stress are recognized as major factors in producing illness. Strife potentially exists in every realm of life: work, play, family, education, community. Intrapersonal and interpersonal conflicts are often compounded by environmental factors seemingly beyond our control (air pollution, threat of warfare, economic recession). The self-aware individual, with the assistance of health team members, strives to identify conflicts and bring harmony into one's lifestyle. The holistic health movement, recognizing the role of the environment, promotes the "regeneration of society in such a way as to foster the optimum health of its members."[9]

8. Utilization of a person's spiritual resources or belief structure is an important aspect of the holistic healing process.

Regardless of an individual's specific spiritual or religious faith, this element can make an important contribution to healing if fully utilized. As one proponent observes: "The structure of an individual's personal belief system concerning the nature of himself and his universe governs the person's experience."[10]

There appears to be a strong relationship between the premises underlying holistic health and those underlying the field of leisure and therapeutic recreation. Certainly, both espouse similar basic beliefs when therapeutic recreation is conceptualized from a humanistic, holistic, social-system perspective. Ample evidence abounds that some recreation therapists are currently using techniques that are compatible with holistic health practices. For example, the use of visual imagery in treating pain and in caring for terminally ill patients is employed to encourage relaxation. And practitioners typically attempt to tap a person's innate strengths and capacities in helping them learn to cope and to develop skills. Further, because recreation often takes place in social settings (recall our earlier mention that social interaction is the chief motive for leisure participation), groups are a primary vehicle used within the profession.

But to what extent exactly is therapeutic recreation part of the holistic health movement? First, it is important to acknowledge that while there is substantial public and professional support for this model, it cannot yet be considered a dominant service model, at least in terms of the number of facilities and practitioners in the profession. Second, in existing holistic health settings, therapeutic recreation has not played an active role. In light of the strong relationship between the two, this phenomenon is extremely unfortunate. The reasons for this are numerous. Play and other forms of healthy human expression may be encompassed by allied practices, such as "stress reduction," "music and sound in health," and so on. Perhaps therapeutic recreators have not been assertive enough or have not articulated the value of their services and how these can be integrated within a holistic framework. A third reason, offered as a critique of the profession, may be that therapeutic recreation has accepted the medical model to the near exclusion of other models. Perhaps, also, therapeutic recreators simply have not seen themselves in a holistic healing context.

However, this does not mean that the hitherto low profile of therapeutic recreation in holistic health will not change. As Otto and Knight state:

> Emerging today is a refreshing openness, an eagerness and willingness by practitioners to learn from the experience of others in the health sciences and the broad field of healing. This openness to new ideas and approaches distinguishes an increasing number of contemporary professionals and practitioners in the field of healing.[11]

THE TEAM APPROACH

> Teamwork is that work which is done by a group of people who possess individual expertise, who are responsible for making individual decisions, who hold a common purpose, and who meet together to communicate, share and consolidate knowledge, from which plans are made, future decisions are influenced and actions are determined.[12]

The *team approach* is another reflection of the holistic health delivery system. Fast becoming accepted as a sound approach to most clinical services, the team is composed of individuals with various types of professional training and expertise who work together as a unit to assist an individual in seeking health and maximum functioning. The "team" that works with a given individual will vary in membership as a function of the specific setting in which services are being delivered (for example, psychiatric hospital, physical disability rehabilitation center, acute pediatric unit of a hospital), and as a function of the problems being experienced by the individual.

Multidisciplinary or Interdisciplinary Team

Most rehabilitation settings tout the concept of the *interdisciplinary* team. This refers to a

functioning unit, composed of individuals with varied and specialized training, who coordinate their activities to provide services to a client or group of clients.[13]

The application of this concept is currently practiced in diverse settings, including child abuse treatment, corrections, education, treatment of chronic and long-term care patients, and community mental health.

The working of an interdisciplinary team is based upon the assumption that the human organism is dynamic, is an integrated whole, and the treatment must be dynamic and fluid in order to keep pace with the changing person.[14] The team recognizes that a given presenting problem cannot be treated in isolation. Take, for example, an individual who is in rehabilitation as a result of a heart attack (myocardial infarction). The physical condition could well be a result of a high-stress job, poor nutrition, a passive leisure lifestyle, and/or a failing marriage. In addition to treating the physical condition, the team would be available to assist the individual in enacting behavioral changes, learning new patterns for coping with stress, and working on interpersonal concerns.

This time-consuming effort requires constant communication among team members, a sharing of knowledge and skills, and often a stepping out of traditional roles to cross profession-to-profession boundaries. The efforts of the team are as much a result of unique personal qualities and skills on the part of each team member as they are on the members' professional training. Ideally, team members support and respect each other's contribution in enabling the patient to attain maximum independence.

For example, a rehabilitation nurse might become part of the team headed on a recreational outing (a weekend ski trip) to ensure that someone is available to administer medications and treat medical emergencies. On the other hand, a therapeutic recreator with counseling skills might co-lead a psychotherapy group. This approach demands that the workers minimize professional jealousies and maximize the strengths of each team member.

The most important participant on the team is the patient, or health seeker. The more the individual is able and is expected to participate in his or her own recovery, the more speedy the recovery is apt to be. Insofar as it is feasible, the individual is presented with meaningful treatment alternatives. The resulting course of action will then be based somewhat on personal decisions as well as upon prescription.

In reality, the interdisciplinary concept is difficult to put into practice. Often, what is manifested is a multidisciplinary concept, which utilizes the efforts of appropriate disciplines but without a great deal of skill sharing among professionals. Each professional maintains a more or less traditional role (according to training) in the treatment process.

The role and actual tasks performed by the therapeutic recreator will vary. In a rehabilitation function, therapeutic recreators help others to understand the importance of recreation, play, and leisure in life; its impact on the overall quality of life; its relationship to self-confidence, perceived competence, coping, and motivation; its importance within healthy family functioning and within the fabric of community life.

PSYCHOSOCIAL FACTORS IN REHABILITATION

In Chapter 5, the reader was introduced to the psychosocial aspects of disability. The following section of this chapter will elaborate on selected psychosocial factors that are particularly relevant to therapeutic recreators with rehabilitation functions. Each of these factors (along with others) is considered in developing and implementing programs and services.

Self-Perceptions

How individuals perceive themselves seems to be a critical factor in the success of rehabilitation efforts. Ample evidence suggests that a primary focus of the professional's role within rehabilitation is to increase the patient's positive self-perceptions. Given multiple social or environmental cues that it is not acceptable to be ill or disabled, this effort on the part of the professional takes on increased significance.

Learned Helplessness

Helplessness is the psychological state that frequently results when events, behaviors, and their outcomes are perceived as uncontrollable. That is, when a person's efforts have no effect on events or behaviors, helplessness is inferred. The person experiencing this state might say, "It makes no difference what I do, I can't change anything." Helplessness, then, is not an inherent human characteristic; rather, it is learned.[15]

If one believes that he or she is helpless or powerless, motivation to reach goals or to succeed is greatly minimized. Iso-Ahola suggests, then, "that the main task of the [recreation] therapist is to increase the patient's perceived control and mastery over the environment and to prevent them from inferring helplessness."[16] Of course, some events are uncontrollable by the individual. Therefore, it is helpful for the patient to be able to discriminate between events that can be controlled and those that cannot. Naturally, individuals differ in the degree of perceived helplessness or sense of personal control.

Implications in therapeutic recreation. It is expected that individuals can be assisted to decrease perceived helplessness and to increase a sense of personal control. Niles, Ellis, and Witt[17] suggest programmatic directions to assist in this process. These have been adapted and are presented below:

1. In a group, mix "helpless" individuals with more competent individuals.
2. Offer meaningful choices "within" activities.
3. Provide the individual with choices "between activities" that are of equal attractiveness.
4. Offer individual activities in which participants have equal possibilities for success and failure.
5. Increase the individual's skills and knowledge base through leisure education (see Chapter 12).
6. Offer skills to be learned that are of specific interest to the individual.
7. Reinforce an individual's abilities and efforts during his or her first encounter with an activity.
8. Winning and losing in competition should not be emphasized.
9. To initiate participation, offer an easy decision, then give details.
10. In situations of failure, tell the individual that his or her failure was caused by a need for more effort or for redirected effort.
11. Be aware that your own perception of an individual's freedom may not be the same as that person's own perception of freedom.
12. In successful situations, remind the participant that perseverance and practices paid off!

For a more in-depth discussion of these guidelines, the reader can refer to the *Leisure Diagnostic Battery: Background, Conceptualization and Structure* (see reference to Niles, Ellis, and Witt at end of this chapter).

Sick Role and Dependency

While most of us do not enjoy being even temporarily sick, we are nonetheless aware of its advantages. (What student hasn't feigned illness just once to delay the responsibility of turning in an assignment? We can even think ourselves into being "under the weather.")

> That there are particular privileges reserved for those with physical or mental impairment can probably most easily be recognized by recalling the privileges you had as a child when you were sick. . . .
> Meals were brought to me in bed.
> I didn't have to go to school.

I had the first choice of the toys.
I was exempt from doing the dishes . . .
I had fresh orange juice or chicken soup or . . . [18]

Does that conjure up some warm feelings? Talcott Parsons, in describing the "sick role," identified two characteristics: (1) exemption from social responsibility and (2) release from expectation of taking care of self.[19] Whereas an occasional sickness may be psychologically healthy (it gives us time to think, to reflect; offers an opportunity to reexamine lifestyle, choices, life patterns, and so forth), some individuals may have a difficult time letting go of the sick role. This interferes with successful rehabilitation. In other instances, the sick role may be supported (often unconsciously) by elements within the rehabilitation system, creating detrimental dependence.

Implications.   Professionals monitor their relationship with patients and clients to determine if unnecessary dependence is developing on the part of either party. The art and science of creating healthful, helpful interactions is beyond the scope of this book. However, therapeutic recreators recognize dependency as a major consideration in rehabilitation efforts because consumers are often particularly vulnerable and can become overly dependent.

Perceptions of Deviance

In an earlier chapter we discussed ways of minimizing the perceptions a disabled individual has or that others have of devalued differentness—or deviance. Because rehabilitation services are often based on the medical model with its inherent focus on illness, it is particularly important for therapeutic recreation specialists to be cognizant of the potential effects of operating in this system. Through the provision of services which are sensitive to this issue, the client can be assisted in remaining attuned to his or her "acceptable" self (i.e., self-esteem).

Implications: normalizing programming.   Programs based upon the concept of normalization use activities, settings, and strategies that are as close as possible to being typical and socially valued. The following guidelines are based upon the writings of Wolfensberger,[20] and Hutchison and Lord.[21]

1. The settings used are the same or as similar as possible to those used by nondisabled individuals. Whenever possible, strive to use community settings used by the public.
2. Activities approximate those in which nondisabled persons of the same age engage. Activities are diverse enough to provide opportunities for decision making, risk taking, with the possibility of experiencing both success and failure. Whatever the experiences available, they facilitate real play and leisure behavior.

In some rehabilitative settings that serve persons who are severely mentally retarded or mentally ill, adults will function at a much younger developmental age. It is important that recreation personnel recognize the developmental stage or the "entry level" of the person: For example, you would not attempt to engage an individual in a game using a complex set of rules who has not yet been successful with games with simpler rules. You might, however, adapt a complex game so that it could be played using simpler rules. "Duck, duck, goose" or any other children's game is inappropriate for an adult, regardless of their developmental level. In any situation, the individual is accorded dignity and respect.

3. Because clinical or medical-sounding labels tend to reinforce disability and illness and increase the image of deviance/differentness, use titles to reflect the intent of the program.

Losses and Grief

Patients may experience many different kinds of losses. A loss of a part of the body or of physical, mental, or emotional function will no doubt be the antecedent that led the individual to the use of rehabilitation services. Other potential losses include: loss of body image; losses associated with hospitalization (loss of private space; loss associated with dependence on others for dressing oneself and other intimate functions); loss of control; loss of certainty about the future, in relationship to personal health and independence, and in relationship to loved ones; and loss in relationship to lifestyle. In the case of terminally ill patients, the individual is dealing with the loss of his or her own life.

Typically, these types of losses will result in the person going through the grief process, which parallels that described by Elisabeth Kubler-Ross in her classic study on death and dying.[22] She identified five stages in this process: (1) denial and isolation; (2) anger; (3) bargaining; (4) depression; and (5) acceptance.

Implications for services. Professionals will learn to recognize the manifestations of these stages of grieving. Certainly, they will be sensitive to individuals at every stage and recognize that different types of responses are needed at each level. Often a good listening ear and a "shoulder" are the most important contributions that a therapeutic recreator can offer. Our effectiveness as a listener is likely to be enhanced if we ourselves have attempted to deal with death and grieving. Because this role is personally draining, professionals may need their own support system to help them deal with the demands of an environment in which people are dying.

Medications

Although not strictly a psychosocial factor, the use of medications with patients has varied implications in programming. The reader is urged to become familiar with medications used in various rehabilitation settings because certain kinds of activities (food-related; activities in the sun or in the water, for example) may be contraindicated. Further, therapeutic recreators can play a vital role in helping doctors adjust doses of medicine by being alert to mood and energy changes of patients.

Social Networks

Significant others cannot be ignored in rehabilitation services. Certainly the existence of a severe illness or disability will affect the family or peer network of the patient. Thus, researchers stress the importance of the family or significant others in creating a supportive environment and in contributing to the motivation for success.[23]

Implications. Service providers cannot make assumptions about *who* an individual's "significant others" are. It is the individual who determines how significant specific persons are to him or her.[24] Therapeutic recreators can help find ways of counteracting the isolation often caused by hospitalization by using networks that are meaningful to the individual.

Swenson suggests that interventions, using networks, can follow two directions: (1) engaging existing networks and seeking to enhance their functioning and (2) creating new networks that help link formerly isolated individual to groups.[25] One strategy used for "mapping" networks, showing the number and intensity of relationships that a person possesses, is illustrated in Figure 11-1.

In this example, those individuals within the circle have a relatively close or intimate relationship with the client; those outside the circle have a

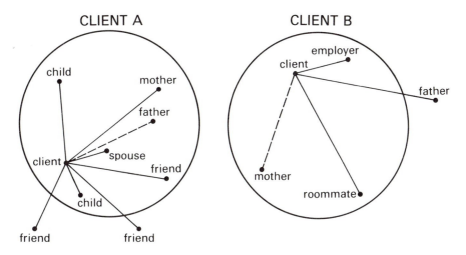

FIGURE 11-1 Mapping Social Support Networks

less close relationship, but have (had) some influence on the client. Broken lines connect to deceased persons.

Using Figure 11–1, we see that clients A and B have very different social support systems. With client A, the therapeutic recreator may attempt to mobilize these significant others (as perceived by the client) to help in the rehabilitation efforts. For example, he or she may encourage these individuals to use recreation activities to help the client achieve success in reaching a goal.

Another form of social networks is found within self-help groups, which have grown considerably in recent years. Self-help groups generally consist of two major categories of individuals: (1) those with certain conditions who have experienced common personal or social inequities, as represented by Alcoholics Anonymous and People First, and (2) family members or friends of individuals with common experiences, such as Friends Outside or Alanon. The growth in the number and types of self-help groups in both the United States and around the world has been impressive. Recovery, Inc. (a mental health support group), Alcoholics Anonymous, and the Boston Self-Help Center are only three examples of organizations whose membership assumes responsibility for planning, implementing, and evaluating services for its members—all of whom have one kind of disability or another.

Peer relationships are central to the effectiveness of the model. Peers who share common conditions work together to effect change in themselves and others. Each member has a status equal to other members and can assume a share of ownership for the change that occurs.

Professionals tend to have a peripheral role, if any, within this model. However, therapeutic recreators have been known to be active promoters of this concept and have facilitated the development of such groups by helping to provide meeting space and identifying community resources.

Further, therapeutic recreators are generally aware of the existence of such groups in specific communities and can help link recently disabled persons with these groups. The group can provide support as the individual makes a transition from the clinical to the community setting.

THE RELATIONSHIP BETWEEN REHABILITATION AND THE ENVIRONMENT

The assumption underlying the specialized environment is that just as certain environments are commonly acknowledged to be detrimental to health, other environments will be therapeutic for certain individuals. If these individuals spend a given period of time in the specially designed environment, they will come out "better." Their improvement may be subjective in that they will feel better or believe they have progressed; and/or it may be objective in that those observing them will judge them to have improved. The area of improvement might be physical—increased strength, stamina, range of motion or coordination—or it may be psychological and emotional—relief of anxiety, depression, fear, confusion or a decrease in craving for substances such as drugs and alcohol. The improvement might also be social or moral—an increased willingness to conform to the laws of a community or to fulfill the roles of a social group, or to adhere to religious principles and practices.[26]

The process of rehabilitation is complex, involving not only a rehabilitation of the body and/or mind but also a revival of the spirit.[27] The process is further complicated because individuals/patients are often faced with the irreversibility of the effects of a debilitating disease or the sudden onset of disability. This personal change affects self-esteem, social relationships, personal identity, and feelings about the future; it also poses a confrontation with seemingly insurmountable environmental barriers. Reflecting the ecological perspective, Brodsky and Platt state:

> Because rehabilitation deals with function and not with symptoms and because each human being functions in a social and psychological as well as physical setting, the person-environment fit is crucial.[28]

This point is reiterated by Edwin Wilhems, then a psychologist at the Texas Institute for Rehabilitation and Research. He suggested that, because the onset of disability disrupts an individual's daily repertoire of behavioral performances, the "central problems of rehabilitation cluster around performance and environment."[29] He states:

> Rehabilitation comprises programmatic arrangements designed to restore or substitute as much as possible a person's lost or altered repertoire, to teach him new forms of performance and new kinds of relations to the environment and to alter environments in appropriate ways.[30]

This perspective is put into practice when a therapeutic recreation staff from a physical rehabilitation facility takes a small group of patients on a weekend ski trip. During this outing, the individual can use adaptive ski equipment to participate in activities that were enjoyed prior to the onset of the disability. In addition, the individuals may experiment with getting around motels, restaurants, and other public facilities. They also may confront stares and other reflections of public attitudes. Elements of the environment that may be specifically adapted include transportation and ski equipment. General concerns include looking for architecturally accessible facilities. The individual also has the opportunity to experiment with various behaviors in response to these environmental elements.

Nursing or convalescent homes and their effects on the health of residents have been the focus of extensive study.

> That environmental characteristics do have a significant effect on adaptation (of residents) to new surroundings, consequent to institutional relocation, is now sufficiently well documented to be accepted.[31]

Lieberman is quoted in the review of research in this area:

> . . . facilitative environments were those characterized by relatively high degrees of autonomy, fostering personalization of the patients, and community integration. Critical was that facilitative environments placed the locus of control much more in the hands of the patient, differentiating among them and permitting them a modicum of privacy.[32]

Skilled nursing facilities often employ therapeutic recreators to work in "activity departments." Practitioners can go beyond the provision of activities by providing the environmental elements suggested above as part of the program offered. For example, providing meaningful activity choices can foster decision making and, in turn, give residents some control over their immediate environment. Encouraging residents to share with other residents and staff the skills they possessed in their preinstitutionalized life can further lead to a sense of personal competence and control. Frequent outings to the community can help minimize isolation from the mainstream of life.

Therapeutic recreators share the responsibility not only to draw people out of the social recesses but also to design an environment that taps individual vitalities. Again, remember that observed behavior is often influenced by the nature of the environment. Thus, the impoverished environments in which some persons (elderly and disabled) find themselves camouflages enormous human riches, wisdom, and ability. Enriching environments help reveal personal dignity.

POTENTIAL GOALS WITHIN REHABILITATION

Based upon the preceding discussion, the following are suggested as goals within therapeutic recreation services:

1. To increase awareness of personal feelings.
2. To assist in the adjustment to the onset of disability or illness.
3. To facilitate successful transition through the grieving process.
4. To strengthen physical adaptive behaviors.
5. To increase personal confidence in selected activities.
6. To increase personal confidence in interacting with social peers.
7. To increase the degree to which the individual attributes personal success to his/her own actions.
8. To increase mastery over getting around independently in one's community.
9. To increase perceived competence in selected behaviors.
10. To increase appropriate expression of feelings.
11. To increase one's sense of self-esteem.
12. To strengthen individuals' interpersonal bonds with significant people (family members, friends).

13. To facilitate successful transition to the home and community.
14. To assist in increasing the responsiveness (physical, social, emotional support) of the home environment to the individual.

These are only suggested programmatic goals. The selected goals of any therapeutic recreation rehabilitation program will be based on the agency within which it is housed, the people served, the conditions of the environment to which the patient/client is returning (if the rehabilitative program is short-term), and related variables.

Further, individual goals and objectives will be based upon the individual (refer to Chapter 10) in collaboration with the therapist.

COMMUNITY-BASED APPROACHES TO REHABILITATION

Prevention

The *preventative* approach is closely allied with the holistic health movement. This approach is based upon consumer self-awareness and education regarding the possible disease-oriented implications of destructive behaviors and environments. Nowhere is this preventative model better suited than with elderly persons "at risk" of becoming institutionalized. Alternative, community-based programs called Adult Day Health are a means used to assist elderly individuals to cope with new life conditions (loss of loved ones, loss of adequate income, loneliness). Preventative services offer continuity in lifestyle and encourage individuals to utilize their personal capabilities.

Community Mental Health Treatment

Community-based mental health programs evolved as a part of the deinstitutionalization process in the 1960s, and the movement is related primarily to the fields of mental health and mental retardation. The major premise underlying this model was the need for a full range of services that would assist individuals in need and the preference for community living over institutional living. One of the major concerns facing consumers and providers alike was the response of the community to community-based services and to the clientele of the services. As a result, many of these services were located in the poorer sections of the community. In some areas, large disability "ghettos" developed. In many communities, these individuals are virtually homeless.

Researchers have theorized that the response or attitude of society to persons with disabilities may be critical in sustaining the mental health of these people. Hence, the need to influence the public's attitude in a positive way has become another mission of many of those working in rehabilitation.

Changes in Health Care Delivery

Compare for a moment two health care settings. One is a typical hospital environment in which an individual is dying from a lengthy illness. The room is shared by two or more patients who are strangers to each other until they are given their room assignments. The room itself is white and furnished with beds having heavy metal siderails, a few chairs, and bedside stands. A medicinal odor envelops the room and adjoining hallway. The door is open, and strangers passing by occasionally peer in. The dying individual sees her family and friends during prearranged visiting hours; otherwise, personal contact is limited to sometimes uncomfortable medical procedures performed by caring but overworked personnel.

If this institution is fortunate enough to employ therapeutic recreators or social workers, it may be these people who provide time for talking, sharing, and needed emotional support. The likelihood that the patient will have a sense of personal control, dignity, and respect in this environment is limited.

An alternative to the hospital environment is the hospice movement, which is growing in popularity. Emerging from the holistic healing movement, the hospice movement strives to provide a dignified and nurturing environment that will assist both the dying individual and his or her family. It offers not only physical facilities (a natural, homelike, and private environment) but also health and human services that respond to the physical, emotional, social, and spiritual state of the individuals comprising the family or other significant social unit.

As of now, therapeutic recreators are not often employed as part of the professional team within hospice settings. But as the value of play as a healthy and lifelong human experience becomes increasingly recognized, therapeutic recreators will undoubtedly play a more active role in these services.

This comparison is meant to point out that professionals are becoming increasingly aware of environmental considerations in every part of life and, as a result, major service delivery systems are undergoing massive changes.

The Rehabilitation of Society

There should be little doubt about the important role "society" assumes in the overall well-being of individuals. The focus of rehabilitation, then, must include the community as well as the individual. This concept will be developed in Chapter 13.

PROFESSIONAL ISSUES FOR THERAPEUTIC RECREATION IN REHABILITATION

Rapidly escalating medical costs, combined with consumer and funder demand for accountability, have caused therapeutic recreators to become even more concerned with the delivery of quality services. Specific issues such as cost-effectiveness, efficacy of services (that is, what was their impact?), the documentation of who was served, for how long, by whom, and individual patient results have been addressed at the local, state, and national levels.

Quality Assurance

Accrediting agencies, such as the Joint Commission on Accreditation of Hospitals (JCAH) and the Commission on Accreditation of Rehabilitation Facilities (CARF), have established standards to which service providers wishing to be recognized through accreditation are expected to conform. Standards have been set for most rehabilitation settings, such as psychiatric, alcoholism, and drug abuse facilities; hospitals; long-term care facilities; and community mental health service programs.

The standards set by the accrediting agency include criteria for many aspects of service delivery: scope of services (orientation, program content); the existence of program objectives; the implementation of individual program or treatment plans; documentation of services; the scheduling of services; and administrative concerns, such as staff composition and supervision, and continuing education. These standards apply to all services available within the provider agency.

Further, the National Therapeutic Recreation Society (NTRS) developed its own standards devoted specifically to therapeutic recreation services. Therapeutic recreators will continually work to upgrade their services not only to meet but to surpass these minimum-level requirements. The intent of these standards is to continuously upgrade the quality of health care services. However, standards are still in the developmental stage and thus actual service delivery in rehabilitation settings still tends to vary widely.

Third-Party Reimbursement

Growing economic stresses require that departments within medical settings justify their services and expenditures. There is pressure from administrators of facilities that services be at least partially reimbursable or self-supporting. That is, rather than the hospital subsidizing services, departments are encouraged to find other sources of support. The "bill" for services may be paid directly by the consumer (which is very rare in this age of expensive medical care), paid by a third party, such as the government (through Medicare, Medicaid), or by a private sector insurance company, such as Blue Cross/Blue Shield or Aetna.

Obtaining reimbursement for services is difficult; many factors complicate the receiving of financial coverage. Different insurers use different reimbursement categories and criteria. Diagnostic-related groups (DRGs) have been developed as one basis for categorizing medical conditions for purposes of financial coverage.

Third-party reimbursement generally requires that nationally accepted standards of practice be in effect. As indicated earlier, although great strides have been made in this effort, nationally accepted standards in therapeutic recreation have not yet been fully implemented.

Representatives from state professional organizations and NTRS have worked closely with third-party reimbursers in order to have "therapeutic recreation services" written into regulations and accreditation services. Particularly important is interaction with the federal government, through the Social Security Act. Professionals in the field can expect this to remain a critical issue through the 1980s and 1990s.

SUMMARY

This chapter emphasized the nature of therapeutic recreation within the context of rehabilitation: its service models; purpose; its consumers; its environments; and its practices. Although this chapter is only introductory (rehabilitation is very complex and involves many factors, too many to acknowledge here), the authors intended to present broad parameters of rehabilitation. The reader is reminded that it is erroneous and dangerous to examine issues or activities in isolation of one another. Therefore, we attempted to link several of the aspects of rehabilitation together to present a more unified picture. Rehabilitation professionals need to respond sensitively to the client/patient and to recognize the patient's critical physical and social environments.

DISCUSSION QUESTIONS

11-1.   Define rehabilitation in your own words. What services are often a part of the rehabilitation process?

11-2.   How can therapeutic recreation contribute to the rehabilitation process?

11-3.   Compare the medical and holistic health models. How are they similar? How do they differ?

11-4.   Discuss the similarities of the holistic health model and the ecological perspective of therapeutic recreation.

11-5.   What does it mean to have a "team approach"?

11-6.   There are several psychosocial factors that need to be addressed in a rehabilitation setting. The factors are listed below. For each, what is the implication for therapeutic recreation?
learned helplessness
sick role
deviance
losses and grief

medications
·social networks

Why are therapeutic recreators concerned with these factors? That is, what is the relationship of these factors to leisure?

11-7. What are potential rehabilitation goals within therapeutic recreation?

CASE STUDY

This activity is to be conducted in groups of two to three students per group. Each group is to simulate a therapeutic recreation staff within a rehabilitation hospital.

The hospital's administration, faced with rising hospital costs and limits in funding, is conducting an assessment of each department functioning within the setting. The administration is asking each department to provide it with a solid rationale and justification for its continued existence within the hospital. Specifically, it is asking for:

an explanation of how your department contributes to the overall rehabilitation of the individual
what specific needs of the individual the staff addresses
the general treatment goals of the department
an evaluation of the overall effectiveness of the staff
a plan for documenting the individual progress of each patient served
any other information you think will contribute to your justification

Within your group, you are to develop a rationale for your therapeutic recreation program, responding to the specific items listed above.

Note:

Articulating the role of therapeutic recreation may be one of the most important tasks of the professional, regardless of the setting. You may want to contact the local therapeutic recreation staff of a rehabilitation center to gather more insight into how they explain what therapeutic recreation contributes in that type of environment.

NOTES

[1]Robert J. Flynn and Kathleen E. Nitsch, eds., *Normalization, Social Integration, and Community Services* (Baltimore· University Park Press, 1980), p. 4.

[2]Robert M. Goldenson, ed., *Disability and Rehabilitation Handbook* (New York: McGraw-Hill, 1978), p. 8.

[3]Gerald O'Morrow, *Therapeutic Recreation: A Helping Process,* 2nd ed. (Reston, Va: Reston Publishing Co., 1980), p. 168.

[4]Scout Lee Gunn and Carol Ann Peterson, *Therapeutic Recreation Program Design: Principles and Procedures* (Englewood Cliffs, N.J., Prentice-Hall, 1978), pp. 15, 111.

[5]Arthur C. Hastings, James Fadiman, and James S. Gordon, eds., *Health for the Whole Person* (Boulder, Colo.: Westview Press, 1980), p. 3.

[6]Herbert Otto and James Knight, eds., *Dimensions on Wholistic Healing: New Frontiers in the Treatment of the Whole Person* (Chicago: Nelson-Hall, 1979), p. 3.

[7]Ibid., pp. 8–13.

[8]Ibid., p. 9.

[9]Ibid., p. 12.

[10]Kenneth R. Pelletier, "Mind as Healer and Mind as Slayer," *Lifelong Learning*, September–October, 1975, pp. 1–3.

[11]Otto and Knight, *Wholistic Healing*, p. 5.

[12]Naomi I. Brill, *Teamwork: Working Together in the Human Services* (Philadelphia: J.B. Lippincott, 1976), p. XVI.

[13]Alex J. Ducanis and Anne K. Golin, *The Interdisciplinary Health Care Team: A Handbook* (Germantown, Md.: Aspen Systems, 1979), p. 3.

[14]Ibid., p. 4.

[15]Seppo Iso-Ahola, *The Social Psychology of Leisure and Recreation* (Dubuque, Iowa: Wm. C. Brown, 1980), p. 328.

[16]Ibid., p. 323.

[17]Sharon Niles, Gary Ellis, and Peter A. Witt, "Attribution Scales: Control, Competence, Intrinsic Motivation," in *The Leisure Diagnostic Battery: Background, Conceptualization and Structure*, eds. Gary Ellis and Peter Witt (Denton, Tex.: North Texas State University, Division of Recreation and Leisure Studies, 1981), pp. 28–32.

[18]Ruth Purtillo, *The Allied Health Professional and the Patient: Techniques of Effective Interaction* (Philadelphia: W.B. Saunders, 1973), p. 49.

[19]Talcott Parsons, *The Social System* (Glencoe, Ill.: Glencoe Illinois Free Press, 1951), pp. 436–437.

[20]Wolf Wolfensberger, *The Principle of Normalization in Human Service* (Toronto, Ontario: National Institute on Mental Retardation, 1975).

[21]Peggy Hutchison and John Lord, *Recreation Integration* (Ottawa, Ontario: Leisurability Publications, Inc., 1979), pp. 51–75.

[22]Elisabeth Kubler-Ross, *On Death and Dying* (New York: Macmillan Publishing Co., 1969).

[23]Russell L. Malone, "Expressed Attitudes of Families of Aphasics," in *Social and Psychological Aspects of Disability*, ed. Joseph Stubbins (Baltimore: University Park Press, 1977), pp. 97–102.

[24]Iso-Ahola, *Social Psychology of Leisure and Recreation*, pp. 1–17.

[25]Carol Swenson, "Social Networks, Mutual Aid, and the Life Model of Practice," in *Social Work Practice*, ed. Carel B. Germain (New York, N.Y.: Columbia University Press, 1979), pp. 213–238.

[26]Carroll M. Brodsky and Robert T. Platt, *The Rehabilitation Environment* (Lexington, Mass.: D.C. Heath & Co., 1978), p. 1.

[27]Ibid., p. 3.

[28]Ibid., p. 4.

[29]Edwin P. Willems, "Behavioral Ecology and Health Status and Care," in *Human Behavior and Environment: Advances in Theory and Research*, eds. Irwin Altman and Joachim Wohlwill (New York, N.Y.: Plenum Press, 1976), p. 215.

[30]Ibid., p. 215.

[31]Kermit Schooler, "Environmental Change and the Elderly," in *Human Behavior and the Environment: Advances in Theory and Research*, eds. Irwin Altman and Joachim F. Wohlwill, Vol. 1 (New York: Plenum Press, 1976), pp. 265–298.

[32]M.A. Lieberman, "Relocation Research and Social Policy," *The Gerontologist*, 14 (1974), 494–501.

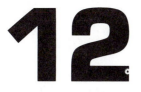

EDUCATING FOR LEISURE EXPRESSION AND SOCIAL INTEGRATION

During the evaluation of a 12-week social development program, the therapeutic recreation staff of a municipal recreation department discussed their frustration with the program. They noted that the same people returned to the program each time it was offered, but they seemed to make no noticeable gains in the acquisition of skills. For example, they noted that Susan still relied on the staff to make decisions for her; George remained on the periphery of the group and never initiated contact with other participants. The staff believed that the program was somewhat repetitious in the activities presented but also believed that most participants enjoyed the activities anyway.

The department director intervened. She first asked the staff to clarify the intended outcomes of the program, then she asked for a careful review of how techniques were selected that would help participants reach these goals. After an analysis of how programs were delivered, the staff discovered that they were putting emphasis on providing activities but did not pay careful attention to strategies that would enable program participants to gain skills. They further recognized that the mere provision of activities does not ensure that participants would gain benefits beyond participation itself. It became apparent that most skills had to be carefully taught in order to ensure learning.

INTRODUCTION

This chapter examines the processes and strategies used in leisure education, the aspect of the service delivery system that emphasizes the development of skills needed to appreciate fully the leisure experience. The second part of the chapter discusses the process of social integration of disabled and able-bodied persons.

One barrier that any individual may face in engaging in leisure pursuits is inadequacy or the absence of skills necessary for participation. The broader an individual's repertoire of social or activity skills, the more likely he or she is to demonstrate enthusiasm or a proclivity for involvement. Likewise, the narrower the range of skills, the more likely the individual is to be isolated and passive. The first part of this chapter discusses the utilization of the educational process in increasing an individual's leisure competence. A major purpose of education is to help the individual recognize leisure potential and to enable participants to assume personal responsibility for leisure behavior. This process, then, affirms every person's potential for learning, for change, for increasing interdependence, and, ultimately, for meeting his or her own needs for recreation and leisure experiences, regardless of personal limitations.

LEISURE EDUCATION

The term *leisure education* carries diverse interpretations. As one major component of Gunn and Peterson's therapeutic recreation model, it refers to the acquisition of social and activity skills and to the increased awareness of self and of leisure resources available to persons with illnesses and disabilities. In a broader context, Mundy and Odum focused on leisure education as a process with application to all individuals.

> It is viewed as a total developmental process through which individuals develop an understanding of self, leisure and the relationship of leisure to their own lifestyles and the fabric of society.[1]

In this context, leisure education is perceived as a noncategorical (not based on the existence of a disability) aspect of service delivery. It can occur in specialized environments, such as rehabilitation centers, special-education schools, or in generic settings, such as the Girl Scouts, the YMCA, or community recreation centers. The recipients may be ill, disabled, or nondisabled; children or young, middle-aged, or older adults, or any combination of individuals. The educational process may be manifested in small-group discussions, individually assigned exercises, or in a recreation activity, where the focus is on attaining new skills or new understandings.

More important than the "form" assumed are the intended outcomes of the processes encompassed by leisure education. Mundy and Odum listed five processes: leisure awareness; self-awareness; leisure skills; decision making; and social interaction. For each of these processes, they have delineated several potential outcomes (see Table 12–1).

TABLE 12-1 The Process and Output of Leisure Education

PROCESS	OUTPUT
Leisure Awareness	An individual who: knows what leisure is identifies a variety of leisure experiences describes the relationship of leisure to his or her life relates leisure to his or her lifestyle relates the relationship of leisure to the quality of his or her life explains the relationship of leisure to the fabric of society
Self-Awareness	An individual who: is satisfied with his or her leisure interest and its scope whose capabilities are compatible with his or her level of aspirations identifies realistic leisure expectations for self identifies elements of quality leisure experiences for self chooses leisure experiences compatible with personal values can modify elements of leisure experiences to be more compatible with his or her own expectations, interests
Leisure Skills	An individual who: uses planning and process skills for leisure can perform basic entry-level skills in a variety of leisure activities has acquired advanced skills for self-selected leisure experiences
Decision Making	An individual who: identifies, gathers, and applies information regarding leisure identifies alternatives and uses them in making decisions related to leisure identifies possible outcomes of leisure choices makes leisure decisions compatible with his or her self-awareness evaluates leisure decisions
Social Interaction	An individual who: identifies and uses types of verbal and nonverbal communications that contribute to leisure goals identifies, selects, and uses patterns of social interaction

Adapted from Jean Mundy and Linda Odum, *Leisure Education: Theory and Practice* (New York: John Wiley & Sons, 1979), pp. 55–56.

These processes are particularly significant for ill or disabled individuals. For example, recall earlier discussions regarding the historical segregation of these persons from a full-range of leisure expressions. Also, remember the implications of congenital disability; that is, an increased possibility of overprotection of children through important developmental years. Opportunities for skill development in a wide range of leisure experiences generally available to other children may have been drastically limited in disabled youngsters. Leisure education, then, provides a vehicle for developing an awareness of leisure activities and resources and for acquiring skills requisite for participation throughout the life span.

Leisure Education and Perceived Competence

Competence (as a result of skill development) in leisure expression promotes self-concept and contributes to the positive perception of the "player" in the mind of observers.[2] Recalling our discussion of attribution theory, we can say that competence can be used as the explanation for leisure participation. This attribution of competence to self on the part of the participant should enhance his or her intrinsic motivation, which is a goal within therapeutic recreation. Leisure education processes that result in competence, then, are a powerful strategy for improving self-concept and for increasing the positive perceptions of observers regarding the "player."

Leisure Education: Its Relationship to Mainstreaming and Normalization

The principle of normalization can be set into motion through leisure education. Skills, norms, and behaviors that are valued by society can be encouraged through the educational model. For example, in a dining situation, individuals may learn appropriate ways of ordering a meal, interacting with dining partners, and paying for dinner in a restaurant. These skills could eventually enable the individual to have successful, more independent, restaurant experiences with friends at a later time. For others, appropriate behavior related to dancing, taking public transportation, attending a concert, or joining a fitness class might be important. Through the educational process, the individual learns ways to minimize negative and devalued differences.

Closely related to the principle of normalization is the concept of *social integration*. It has been suggested that a primary barrier to social integration and interaction is the lack of social skills on the part of some persons with disabilities. The resulting effect has been the continuing isolation of persons without socially adept skills from the mainstream of society. Through leisure education, interactive processes required for successful social relationships can be learned.

As individuals move from dependence toward social interdependence and personal independence, and from segregated to more integrated or community-based alternatives, a knowledge of both resources and of ways to access and enter service systems helps immensely in making the transition. Awareness of personal strengths and successful coping mechanisms also support a transition that can yield positive daily activities and interactions.

The individual who has experienced a wide range of opportunities, who has received honest feedback on behaviors and skills, and who has learned ways of appropriately responding to and adapting to immediate environments is the individual who most likely will be a successful and satisfied leisure participant. Although this aspect of service delivery focuses on leisure within one's lifestyle and life span, the functions and behaviors addressed also affect home life, work life, educational endeavors, and every other aspect of life.

To function competently in daily life activities and within the community is a difficult task for just about everyone, given the pressures and stress of contemporary living. For persons with limited experiences and skills in adapting to home and community expectations, the task can be even more onerous.

Five primary skill areas, along with various subskills, have been identified as requisites for successful transition to community life. Leisure-service personnel will be able to relate directly to many of these areas, which are listed in Table 12–2.

TABLE 12–2 Community Living Skill Areas

I. Fiscal Accountability	G. strangers
A. making change	H. landlords
B. budgeting	IV. Communication
C. banking	A. expressive and receptive language
D. shopping	B. telephone use
E. managing money safely	C. letter writing and mailing
II. Community Mobility	D. gathering information for recreation, business, and other activities
A. pedestrian travel	
B. public transportation	V. Interaction with Establishments
C. driving	A. social agencies
D. bicycling	B. churches
III. Social Interaction	C. schools
A. family	D. businesses
B. friends	E. door-to-door sales
C. neighbors	F. health centers
D. social service workers	
E. creditors	
F. intimates	

From Daniel Close, Larry Irvin, Valerie Taylor, and John Agosta, "Community Living Skills Instruction for Mildly Retarded Persons," in Philip S. Strain (ed.), *Social Development of Exceptional Children* (Rockville, Md.: Aspen Publications, 1982), p. 128.

ticipants should have the opportunity to choose from among a variety of skill and age-appropriate activities.

2. Segregated settings should closely approximate integrated settings. Factors to be included in segregated services to enhance similarity of settings are: the use of the approximate leader-participant ratios as employed in settings with non-disabled persons; the use of the same physical settings used by nondisabled persons; and the use of tasks that are similar in complexity, structure, and novelty to those used in regular programs.

3. The amount of transfer increases when meaningful generalization, rather than specific skills or concepts, are developed. For example, if physical fitness is the goal, Hutchison recommends that the emphasis should be on an holistic approach to health care, including nutrition, mental health, and physical endurance, rather than solely on jogging skills.

4. Specific programs based on play and education models maximize confidence and competence. Both components are essential for integration.

5. Programs should be based on developmental sequencing to promote confidence and competence. Hutchison suggests that principles of developmental programming include the use of individualized skills in evaluating individual progress, and the sequencing of tasks and situations from simple to complex.[5]

Selection of activity skills to be developed are contingent on personal needs, interests, motivations, and aspirations, as well as popular social activities. Some individuals may be hesitant about engaging in some experiences, limited by the fear of the unknown or fear of failure. Skill-development opportunities can be set up to provide the necessary physical and emotional support to counterbalance unsuccessful endeavors. Oftentimes, groups of people entering into a similar, unknown situation provide adequate motivation and group support.

"Outward-Bound" and similar outdoor "risk" experiences that deliberately challenge individuals to go beyond their previous personal limits have been enthusiastically received. People with mental illness, severe physical limitations, mental retardation, and other disabilities have discovered new self-esteem by finding and utilizing previously unknown personal strengths and by forming bonds of trust with other group members. Individuals have climbed mountains, traversed rope courses, and overcome extremely adverse conditions this way.

Activity analysis and modification.   Some recreational endeavors, such as games and physical activities, may initially appear unrealistic for successful involvement by individuals with certain disabilities. The process of *activity analysis* involves breaking down an activity into its basic behavioral requirements necessary for participation. Peterson and Gunn suggest that activities may be divided into physical, cognitive, affective, and social requirements.[6] For example, physical requirements include the body position used (sitting, standing, kneeling), the amount of flexibility, types of movement, and the degree of endurance, speed, strength, and coordination needed to participate. Emotional requirements include the degree (intensity) with which emotions can be expressed and the range of emotions required. The degree of concentration needed, the level of planning and strategy, memory retention, and relationships among concepts are part of the cognitive requirements of activities. Social requirements emphasize the nature of the relationships among participants that an activity requires and the social structure used.

Once an activity's requirements have been identified, those requirements which do not match an individual's ability can be changed to use an existing personal skill. Typically, modifications of activities include lowering of apparatus, reduction in the speed of movement (for example, bounce, rather than throw, the ball), additional verbal or visual cues, and the reduction in the size of playing area. For instance, if an individual has little functional use of his or her hands, but desires to play tennis, the racquet may be attached to the participant's wrist with the aid of an elastic bandage.

When selecting an activity, consider the functional requirements of that activity. What does a person need to be able to do in order to be successful engaging in it? In what ways can it be modified to meet and challenge the abilities of the player? Nearly any activity can be adapted to allow for participation by virtually anyone. Remember that persons with visual impairments can ski, that wheelchair users can climb mountains, that hearing-impaired persons can perform in plays and musicals; given the motivation and opportunity, just about everyone can do anything he or she desires.

The following material, taken from *Closing the Gap: An Inservice Training Manual for Mainstreaming Recreation and Leisure Services,* presents several considerations for modifying activities, and the worksheet presented in Table 12-3 provides the reader with an opportunity to think of specific ways in which activities might be adapted.

General Considerations for Modifying Activities[7]

1. Keep the activity and action as close to the original activity as possible. This will enhance the transfer of the skills learned in the recreation environment to the neighborhood or community.
2. Modify only those parts of the activity that require adapting. Keep the experience challenging but success-oriented. For a wheelchair user, changing the surface on which an active game is played from the grass to the pavement may be the only modification necessary.
3. Individualize the adaptations according to the needs of each player. No two people, even with the same disability, are alike.
4. Think *abilities!* Base adaptations on abilities rather than disability. For example, for participants with limited vision, think about their abilities to touch and hear. Supplement a visually oriented experience with auditory cues to enable everyone to participate.
5. Discuss the potential need for modifications with participants. They may have

TABLE 12-3 Worksheet for Adapting Recreational Experiences

ADAPTING RECREATIONAL EXPERIENCES

1. THE *ENVIRONMENT* IN WHICH THE EXPERIENCE TAKES PLACE

Consider	*Suggestions*
Noise level: Excessive background noise will interfere with the ability of hearing-impaired participants to understand speech and may cause individuals with visual impairments to become disoriented	Minimize background noise by using carpets.
	_____
	_____
	Explain directions prior to going or have activity in a quiet spot
Architectural barriers: may restrict participation of individuals with physical limitations (e.g., steps, surface of ground or floor, heavy doors)	Provide accessible parking, ramps, drinking fountains. . .
	_____
	_____
	_____
	_____

2. *LEADERSHIP:* THE WAY IN WHICH MATERIAL IS PRESENTED AND THE LEADER'S INTERACTION STYLE

Consider	*Suggestions*
Mode of presentation (e.g., oral, written)	Use multisensory approach: visual aids to supplement verbal explanations, demonstrate
Sequencing of directions	Sequence from simple to complex and allow sufficient time for practice at each step
The amount of material presented	For individuals with learning difficulties,
	_____
	_____
	_____
	_____
Distance between speaker and listener	_____
	_____
	_____
	_____

Consider	Suggestions
Size and location of the environment	Check transportation possibilities (e.g., consider bus schedules in relationship to program times; car pools)
	_____
	_____
	Provide quiet areas for individuals to relax and socialize at their own pace
Lighting: adequate lighting is essential to maximize the ability of visually impaired persons to see and to enable hearing-impaired individuals to speech-read	Use contrasting colors on visual displays (e.g., black on white)
	_____
	_____

3. *MATERIALS* OR *EQUIPMENT* USED IN VARIOUS ACTIVITIES

Consider	Suggestions
Size of the equipment	_____
	_____
	_____
	Build up the hand grip with adhesive tape to assist individuals with limited hand control
	Create a small table-size game of tetherball with a broomstick and a small rubber ball in a stocking
Weight of the equipment: lighter equipment allows more time for wheelchair users to maneuver their chairs into place, and makes it easier for a person with limited arm strength to participate	_____
	_____
	_____
	_____
	_____
	_____
Sensory dimensions of the equipment: to include participants with visual or hearing impairments, supplementary input is valuable (refer to Appendix B for sources of commercially available equipment).	Auditory balls can be used for ball games
	_____
	_____
	Use changes in surface texture to denote boundaries

TABLE 12–3 [*Cont.*]

Consider	*Suggestions*
4. THE NATURE OF THE EXPERIENCE: THE RULES, TYPE OF ACTIVITY, OR THE APPROPRIATENESS OF AN ACTIVITY FOR PARTICIPANTS	
Age-appropriateness and interest of the activity	
Difficulty level	
Number of participants	Use concrete examples
	Additional players may need to be added in some situations to reduce the amount of activity for players with respiratory difficulties or low fatigue level
Rules of the game	Participants can sit or walk rather than stand or run
	Use the New Games approach, which challenges participants to create their own games and rules
Social interaction pattern	
	Offer alternatives, challenge participants to demonstrate "How many different ways can you. . .?"

Adapted from Target Access, *Closing the Gap: An Inservice Training Manual for Mainstreaming Recreation and Leisure Services,* San Jose State University (Oklahoma State University: National Clearinghouse of Rehabilitation Training Material, 1983), pp. 176–179.

experienced the activity and developed their own adaptations or have ideas on what could be most useful for them.

6. Involve all participants when possible in becoming aware of the process and value of changing games. This will enhance the likelihood that participants will create their own leisure experiences in the community and be enthusiastic and flexible about making changes to include everyone.

Task analysis. Sometimes we tend to avoid teaching certain skills to individuals because we believe that the skill as a whole is too difficult or complex to learn. One strategy that breaks a skill into small, behavioral segments is called *task analysis*. By sequencing the behavioral segments from easy to difficult or simple to complex, an individual masters one segment at a time. This approach has been found to be very effective in teaching even complex skills. Paul Wehman has done extensive research in the use of task analysis, particularly in the development of play skills with severely and profoundly retarded individuals.[8]

Developmental programming. Task analysis is just one strategy encompassed by a broader service delivery concept termed *developmental programming*. This is really a logical approach to working with individuals through designing opportunities that *build on intact individual strengths and abilities* and recognizing that all individuals learn at their own rate, in response to personal motivations. As a programming basic, we start with the individual's "entry point." This is best accomplished through individual and small-group experiences, which provide meaningful decision-making opportunities for each individual.[9]

Central to effective developmental programming are the therapeutic or teaching strategies that practitioners select. Recognizing that individuals learn in different ways, it is helpful to choose strategies that reflect learning preferences. To better understand this idea, think about the way in which you learn best: through lecture and use of tapes (auditory preference); with the use of visual materials, such as written material, graphs (visual preference); through doing and practicing skills (kinesthetic preference). The recognition of sensory-learning preferences will help the provider tap into the learning channels of the individual. In addition, some people prefer individual to small-group learning experiences. Others may prefer to practice skills in the privacy of home or family environments, while others are more socially inclined from the beginning and may prefer the reinforcement others can provide.

Behavioral techniques are those that focus on either reducing or eliminating certain behaviors or those that develop or maintain behaviors. These have been found effective in enabling severely and profoundly retarded persons to develop skills previously believed unattainable. Wehman and Marchant reported a reduction in the stereotypic behaviors of such persons through an increase of appropriate play skills using behavioral strategies.[10]

Focus on Resource Awareness and Utilization

One of the characteristics of a relatively independent individual is the person's ability to access and utilize resources appropriately. Leisure resources include personal (internal) qualities such as values, motivations, skills, and interests. External resources may be within the home and family, in the neighborhood, or in the larger community and may include both designated leisure settings (theaters, golf courses, pools, parks, recreation centers) and personally determined leisure settings (wherever the person decides to engage in leisure), such as the backyard, street, shopping center, in a field). Cultural values, local mores, and allied geographical, cultural, ethnic, and religious variables each contribute to the type and meaning of resources that have significance for the individual. Resources accessible through state, national, or international travel may also be relevant for the individual.

Through leisure-education processes, professionals can assist individuals in recognizing those resources that are available. Community outings are one method of introducing people to new settings. For many, this will include learning how to get to the site when using public or private transportation, and how to maximize the use of the resource.

This process requires that practitioners be knowledgeable about a vast array of resources in their community. For therapeutic recreators who work in clinical settings where patients come from diverse communities, this is particularly demanding. Under any circumstances, practitioners need to be active in their communities and maintain an active communication network in order to stay current in relation to leisure opportunities and resources. In instances where clients come from other outside communities, the practitioner should try to develop a major contact person within those communities.

Focus on Social Skill Development

Most practitioners interacting with persons with disabilities agree that social isolation is a primary problem. As one researcher observes:

> Almost all exceptional children, regardless of their disability or etiology of that disability, have significant social handicaps. Often, the specific handicap is in the form of skill deficits (e.g., lack of verbal skills, lack of knowledge about how to make friends). It is also true, however, that the *primary* social handicap of many exceptional children rests with negative and biased peer attitudes and behaviors. Of course, most often we are confronted with a situation in which skill deficits interact with negative peer attitudes and behaviors.[11]

This perspective reflects the ecological nature of social systems. That is, one must examine both the *context* and *content* of a situation to target and remediate problem areas.

Readers need only to consider their own social network—including family relationships, intimate friendships, school and/or work colleagues and acquaintances—to recognize the significance of appropriate social interaction skills in successful daily living. The behaviors that evolve into social competence are developed throughout our lifetime. Through diverse experiences, we attain behaviors appropriate to a myriad of environments, learning to relate to others and to socially oriented tasks. As one significant component of our adaptive behavior, social competence has been defined as

> those responses, which within a given situation, prove effective . . . maximize the probability of producing, maintaining or enhancing positive effects for the interactor.[12]

Levels of social interaction.   Social isolation takes several forms. The brief case studies below reflect various levels of skill development and peer acceptance.

> Jenny, age 11, has a limited and sometimes unintelligible vocabulary. She frequently attempts to engage her peers (primarily other disabled youth), but is often ignored or rebuffed. Her behavior is often inappropriate to the situation, and she is often overly aggressive. For example, when several of her peers were listening to pop music on a stereo and dancing informally, she attempted to dance with them by getting in the middle of the group and squeezing others out. When they asked her to go away, she started throwing records.

> Steven attends a regular high school and spends a part of each day in the resource room for learning-disabled students. He is cooperative when asked to work with peers on classroom projects, and other students do talk to him during these activities. He works as a bus boy in a restaurant a few nights per week and is a member of the high school band. He is often seen alone during lunch and free hours at school. At home, he spends much time reading in his room or watching T.V. He does not have any close friends. When asked, he can explain how to introduce himself to people and initiate a conversation. He seldom is observed practicing these skills, however.

Both of these individuals experience a degree of social isolation. Particularly evident is the void in friendships, even though Steven appears marginally accepted by his peers.

Research indicates that children's friendships serve critical functions; children without friends appear to be at risk in terms of peer relationships in later life.[13] Before friendships develop, social acceptance may need to be attained. The body of research pertaining to the social skill correlates of social acceptance tends to fall into three major domains of interpersonal tasks: initiation, social maintenance, and conflict resolution.[14] These are briefly explored below.

Individuals are faced with the need to *initiate* social interactions in school, work, leisure, and other daily environments. As disabled persons move into new parts of the community, these skills will become increasingly important. These are characterized behaviorally by extending a greeting (either verbally or by a handshake), exchanging information, and offering inclusion into a group or activity.[15]

Maintenance skills require a broad range of social skills that enable an individual to continue developing relationships. These skills include behaviors such as effective communication, giving positive attention and approval to others, and being helpful and pleasant.[16]

The third domain is *conflict resolution*. Whenever two or more people interact over a period of time, the potential for conflict arises. Skills such as compromise, negotiation, persuasion, and ignoring can each be effective under selected circumstances.[17] Other characteristics of highly socially accepted (thus, popular) children include being a good sport, acting friendly, and tending to the needs of others.

Because social interaction is a reciprocal process, there seems to be a high probability that positive social behavior will elicit positive responses from the social environment. However, the reverse also appears to be true. Deviant or aversive behaviors are likely to elicit a similar response from family members, peers, and others.[18]

Strategies for facilitating social skill development.   Several authors urge the utilization of a systematic behavioral approach to enable persons to develop adequate social skills. This approach

> refers to procedures that decrease or increase (depending on the goals) the frequency of a selected behavior by systematically arranging environmental events that precede or follow it.[19]

Most behavioral studies reveal that social skills training strategies fall into one of three categories: (1) manipulation of antecedents, (2) manipulation of consequences, or (3) modeling appropriate behavior, either by an authority figure or by a peer confederate.[20] The first category, *manipulation of antecedents*, refers to organizing or structuring conditions that will likely elicit certain desired behaviors. Such antecedents could include the physical design of an activity area that encourages interaction, the availability of socially oriented toys or other play material, or a social environment requiring some verbal interactions.

Behaviors also have *consequences*. Consequences can be designed in such a way to encourage or discourage selected behaviors. A smile, a pat on the shoulder, tokens or other appropriate and deserved rewards are given after the demonstration of predetermined behaviors.

Modeling appropriate behavior has traditionally been undertaken by the teacher, parent, therapeutic recreator, or other authority figure. The use of peers, both in person and on film, has become more widely used in recent years.

In services that aim to foster appropriate social interactions, knowledge of the dynamics of group functioning is essential. Avedon delineated eight interactive processes that can be identified in group dynamics. Each of the processes can limit, influence, or regulate the behaviors of persons involved in the process. Further, he suggests that these patterns appear to be developmental in nature; that is, one must master one pattern, include it in his or her behavioral repertoire, then work on another pattern. These patterns are described below.

> *Intraindividual.* Action taking place within the mind of a person or action involving the mind and a part of the body, but requiring no contact with another person or external object.
>
> *Extraindividual.* Action directed by a person toward an object in the environment, requiring no contact with another person.
>
> *Aggregate.* Action directed by a person toward an object in the environment while in the company of other persons who are also directing action toward objects in the environment. Action is not directed toward one another, and no interaction between participants is required or necessary.
>
> *Interindividual.* Action of a competitive nature directed by one person toward another. This is the first of the true dyadic relationships.
>
> *Unilateral.* Action of a competitive nature among three or more persons, one of whom is an antagonist of it. Interaction is in simultaneous competitive dyadic relationships.
>
> *Multilateral.* Action of a competitive nature among three or more persons, with no one person as an antagonist.
>
> *Intragroup.* Action of a cooperative nature by two or more persons intent upon reaching a mutual goal. Action requires positive verbal and nonverbal interaction.
>
> *Intergroup.* Action of a competitive nature between two or more intragroups. This process is inherent in team games.[21]

Social-sexual development.   Another concern of leisure-service personnel is the social-sexual behavior of some individuals with illnesses or disabilities. The sense of intimacy that results from the exclusive relationship of a "best friend" is considered a prerequisite for a mature, adult love relationship.[22]

For those born with disabling conditions, opportunities for developing such a personal relationship are often limited. Attempts to initiate a sexual relationship may be, at best, awkward, and at worst, totally inappropriate. This can result in rejection, loneliness, even desperation.

A wealth of materials on social-sexual education has been developed to address this important concern. Often therapeutic recreation personnel can work with counselors, educators, or others to provide training. Be aware, though, that any educational program should be developmental in nature and focus on self-awareness, feelings, roles, and behaviors.

The feeling of belonging, of having a sense of connectedness or affiliation with a significant other, be it a group or an individual, is a basic social-psychological need. Therapeutic recreators are in an excellent position to assist individuals in meeting this very personal need through educational opportunities.

SOCIAL INTEGRATION AND INTERACTION

Bob, a therapeutic recreator for United Cerebral Palsy Association, works closely with the local municipal recreation department's staff in providing recreation and leisure services for disabled persons in the community. Recently, the staff has discussed possibilities for integrating programs. Bob and his colleagues have reviewed literature on how to bring persons with and without disabilities together successfully and have contacted some communities that have already started integrated programs. They are philosophically committed to mainstreaming, and have several questions.

How do we attract both populations to integrated programs?
How much should we prepare disabled and able-bodied persons before we start integrating services?
What kinds of programs and services should be integrated?
What kinds of skills/attitudes should people in these services possess?
How do we challenge all participants to attain new skills and find maximum satisfaction through engaging in these programs?

The emergence of persons with disabilities in the community requires that therapeutic recreation specialists and allied leisure-service providers alike acknowledge and address those variables that facilitate the successful social interaction of disabled and nondisabled persons. Be aware, however, that the social integration of the two groups does *not* automatically result in meaningful social interaction. In fact, integrating disabled and nondisabled persons may pose some difficulties. One factor suggested by social psychologists as causing problems is the concept of the disabled person as a "newcomer" to the group. People tend to gravitate to those who are similar to themselves in interests, backgrounds, and values.[23] One plausible reason may be that similar persons are also familiar persons, and one can relate to familiar persons more easily. Instances of dissimilarity and unfamiliarity may involve those with communication disorders, sensory loss, and nontypical behavior.

Several variables that might affect a nondisabled person's attraction toward a disabled person include: (1) the amount of exposure to the disabled person, (2) the nature of the information received from exposure to the disabled person, and (3) content of the exposure.[24] Although the attitudes developed from the first encounter are important in determining the nature of succeeding interaction, it is predicted that increased contact between the disabled and nondisabled could lead to increased liking and reduced prejudice if the context of the contact is positive.[25]

Although contact may facilitate interaction, entry into an already formed group or community is more difficult. The advent of a "newcomer" to a group almost invariably is followed by a process of interpersonal reorientation in which the group as a social frame of reference is automatically altered.[26] "Newcomers" may also pose threats to an already existing group. While an individual newcomer does not have sufficient strength to radically alter the group, a block of newcomers may pose substantial threat.[27] This perspective has implications for the methods and processes selected to facilitate integration.

Manipulation of the environment, that is, designing it to foster successful interaction, is advocated by most researchers and practitioners. In general, social integration is approached either through *forward* integration or *reverse* (back door) integration. The former refers to the integration of an individual with a disability into a setting previously serving able-bodied persons. This occurs, for example, when a person who uses a wheelchair attends a ceramics class offered to the public. Reverse integration draws able-bodied persons into a program previously serving only disabled participants.

Elements to Consider in Encouraging Positive Interaction

Regardless of the approach utilized, a variety of elements ultimately affect the success of interaction efforts. This section will review some of the elements and strategies that research has identified as significant in integration. However, these must be examined with some caution because most research has been undertaken with preschool and school-age children in educational settings.

The physical environment. Fundamental environmental factors, such as the physical, spatial, and organizational features of the activity or programming area, influence the social integration of individuals. For example, the type and nature of equipment and materials will influence who will use them. Some playgrounds are plainly not usable by a segment of children because of inaccessibility. However, different playground models are being developed that should allow all children to participate. Hence, the design of the space affects the groupings of participants using the space.

The social environment. The importance of the social structure and situational context in integration is crucial. A statement issued by the White House Conference on Handicapped Individuals suggests that ". . . dignity, independence and integration into community life are fostered for most of us through the means we use to fulfill various social roles."[28] Equality of participants is thought to play an important role in encouraging meaningful social interaction.

Equalized roles can be fostered by ensuring that all participants have the opportunity to share skills, as well as be the recipient of assistance. A disabled person who constantly is the "helpee" will undoubtedly have great difficulty in assuming a status equal to the consistent "helper." On the other hand, the strengths of all participants can be ascertained and utilized. Nondisabled and disabled "buddies" can help each other in reaching common goals. Perhaps they can assist each other in putting on clown makeup; discuss their knowledge about nature; share secrets, or. . . . The reader can no doubt think up many other ideas.

Another consideration is the role that is inherent in certain games. Take, for example, a baseball game. What different roles can you identify? pitcher, catcher, fielder, batter, runner, scorekeeper. What roles (positions) do players usually clamor for? The answer is obvious: the ones considered to have value and which tend to be the more active or visible positions. Passive positions, such as scorekeeper, carry with them less value. All participants in a game or activity enjoy the opportunity to assume valued roles. Players can rotate positions so that no one individual monopolizes (or gets stuck with) any particular position.

Any leisure or play environment is composed of certain social demands, expectations, and rhythms. To ensure the success of participants in a selected setting, the needs and competencies of the individual should be matched to the environment. For example, a fast-paced, competitive activity program would likely frustrate the efforts of a severely physically disabled person who had not yet mastered wheelchair mobility skills. A program fostering cooperative relationships and allowing people to reach goals at their own pace would be more apt to result in success for this individual at this time.

Program structure and purpose. The review of research on integration shows that the simple placement of disabled and able-bodied persons together will not necessarily result in interaction above a minimal level. Careful structuring of programs can enhance both skill development and social interaction. A developmental approach recognizes the skill level of each individual and sequences learning activities to build upon identified strengths.

The major types of effective program structures include: (1) cooperative programs, (2) peer imitation/modeling programs, and (3) human differences training.

Cooperative programs. Programs such as these challenge individuals to work together toward common goals. The efforts of each member contribute to the acquisition of the goal. Rules provide structure to games and can be designed to optimize cooperation. A rule that requires players either to change teams periodically or to change roles can minimize competition. Similarly, rules requiring that all members of a team take an active role before points are awarded foster cooperation. "New Games" is an excellent approach to playing. That is, rules are adjusted to meet the functional abilities, needs, and interests of the group. Everyone can assume a participatory role and everyone can experience success. The focus is on participation, team spirit, and fun, not on winning or losing. Research has demonstrated that cooperative structure promotes interaction between able-bodied and severely handicapped persons.[29]

Cooperation can also be fostered through creative and mutual problem solving. Professionals can pose exploratory questions to participants to initiate thinking about other ways of accomplishing a task. "If you couldn't hear the music, how could you learn to dance?" "If you couldn't see the boundaries, how would you know where to run?" "In what other ways can you move across the floor?" Participants may find that there are a multitude of alternatives to doing things—and that helps provide a bridge to understanding each other.

Peer imitation. Severely or profoundly retarded persons or those with severe emotional disorders often display inappropriate social behavior, which serves to inhibit successful social interactions with able-bodied peers. As mentioned earlier, one approach to increase appropriate behaviors has been the use of able-bodied peers (confederates) as social skill trainers. These individuals serve as role models, which disabled persons are encouraged to imitate. For example, one recent study indicated that over a period of five weeks, autistic children were playing adequately with peers. The peers, too, seemed very capable of drawing their disabled friends into appropriate playful behavior.[30] Socially adept disabled peers can also serve as models.

Human differences and similarities training. Research indicates that the frequency of interaction between nondisabled and severely disabled people was positively correlated with the level of understanding the able-bodied had of those with severe disabilities.[31] Whereas most of the efforts toward behavior change have been directed toward the disabled population—enabling them to acquire goals previously thought unattainable—it is anticipated that the behavior of able-bodied children could also be changed.

Therapeutic recreators can help individuals learn about human differences and similarities in many ways: audiovisual presentations; having disabled persons discuss their disabilities and adaptations which assist them in daily functioning; and through the use of life-size puppets that have disabilities. Encouraging able-bodied individuals to "try on" disabling conditions through role-playing can help them gain some personal insights. For example, the controlled use of occluders (similar to blindfolds but which more accurately simulate various visual limitations), splints, wheelchairs, and earplugs can be very enlightening. When using this technique, it is absolutely *critical* that the therapeutic recreation specialist *reinforce* the ways in which people with disabilities *accomplish* tasks. The failure to do so can likely result in an undesired end—the role player is left with an impression of disability and the frustration of not being able to accomplish tasks, rather than the impression of ability and successful adaptation.

One very effective way to help individuals better understand disability as a human difference is to have them explore their own differences. For example, they can discuss their own abilities, their daily activities, their food likes and dislikes, among many other personal topics.

Equally as important as identifying personal differences and different ways of doing things is the identification of *similarities* among people. Play tasks, such as cooperative collages, can be structured to help participants explore common likes and interests. Learning desired skills together, such as magic tricks or mime, are a few examples for children's programs. Remember that any experience should be structured such that participants leave with both positive and realistic perceptions of ability.

Personal readiness.   The degree of readiness for integration with which able-bodied and disabled participants enter programs and experiences is likely to have an impact upon initial social interactions. There is no universal agreement among educators and practitioners as to the value or appropriateness of preprogram preparation.

Those opposed to this preprogram preparation fear that too much emphasis is placed on the differences caused by disability. However, because most people tend to be curious about disabilities, this appears to be a feasible way of addressing this curiosity.

On the other hand, disabled persons may lack psychological readiness for integration. Thus, activities that assist them in learning how to handle probing or potentially uncomfortable questions or stares can be useful in diminishing fear or embarrassment.

Readiness of parents.   The attitudes of parents toward integration can often be seen in their children. Educational programs that allow parents to observe, to vent concern, ask questions, and separate fact from myth is one strategy for minimizing negative attitudes. Staff-parent (one-on-one) discussions can also help alleviate concerns on the part of parents both with disabled and able-bodied children. For parents who have able-bodied children, previous contact with persons with disabilities may be virtually nil. Discussion groups led by disabled adults can provide needed understanding. Likewise, parents of children with disabilities may lack trust in the motives and behaviors of able-bodied children. Contact with their parents can help alleviate fears.

Questions about differences are likely to emerge over the course of a program. The therapeutic recreation specialist should acknowledge parents' concerns and display an open attitude and answer questions honestly. The extent of the answer should be determined by the age, maturity, and curiosity level of the inquirer. Staff should serve as important role models in maintaining openness, honesty, and respect.

Terminology. *Terminology* or *labels* assigned to participants or to programs that emphasize disability are not appropriate for promoting positive interactions. Rather, program titles should reflect the purpose (for example, "Learning the Art of Mime") or the content ("Shape Up: Aerobics for Beginners"). Subtitles or program descriptions may indicate that: "The program is for people with varied abilities. Call program office if you have specialized requirements that will enable you to fully participate. Sign-language interpreters available upon request."

Program content. The reader should know by now that activities in and of themselves are less important than what is happening to a person while engaging in the activity. Activities are modalities and they should be treated as such. Naturally, they reflect the nature of a program. Thus, the question of modification of the activity or the equipment required for participation may well arise. A general rule of thumb is to modify only if necessary and only to the degree required to enable individual involvement. Modification should not distort the original intent of the activity. For example, participation in a volleyball game might require a lowered net or the use of a larger, softer ball. Rules pertaining to the number of times the ball can be hit on one side of the net might be changed. However, the main elements of the game remain intact.

Activities should be designed to meet the needs (including novelty, fun, challenge) of all participants. Some games or individualized experiences, such as golf or ceramics, while engaged in within a social grouping, can be individualized to recognize each person's functional level.

Staff attitudes. Although this topic is addressed last in the sequence of variables affecting the success of integration, it is likely the *most important variable*. Research studies in both education and recreation reveal that the *key* to successful integration is the staff, their skills, values, and attitudes. Again, the perception of the staff is a most critical determinant in shaping a program, activity, or experience. A staff member who believes that individuals who are able-bodied and individuals who are disabled can successfully interact as peers will probably design an experience that is programmed for those results. Likewise, a skeptical staff member may set up a program to reflect his or her negative expectations. Inservice training, using a variety of educational formats and involving disabled consumers, is a logical strategy for reexamining basic values and attitudes and for upgrading programming and process skills. Both specialists and generalists can work together to design effective programs. Table 12–4 summarizes the major variables discussed in

TABLE 12-4 Planning Integrated Programs: Variables to Consider in Encouraging Positive Interaction and Maximum Participation

VARIABLES	STRATEGIES
A. STAFF	
beliefs, values	provide inservice training
attitudes	involve consumers, parents
skills	
B. PURPOSE OF EXPERIENCE	
play	focus on recreation/play
learning	focus on skill development
C. ROLES OF PARTICIPANTS	
readiness level	assess level
equalized/balanced roles	identify areas of expertise
share valued play roles	initiate cooperative problem solving
D. ENVIRONMENTAL FACTORS	
physical design	vary design of programs
social environment	recognize and openly value differences
rhythm/demands/	individualize to extent possible
expectations/skills	equalize roles
E. PARTICIPANTS (NONDISABLED AND DISABLED)	
attitudes/values/beliefs/fears	use staff as role models
readiness/acceptance level	support open discussion
F. PARENTS	
attitudes/values/beliefs/fears	use staff as role models
level of readiness	provide open discussion
G. TERMINOLOGY USED (PROGRAM AND PARTICIPANT)	
program	eliminate labels that focus on disability
participant	use terms that reflect function (on titles, on publicity, etc.)
H. ACTIVITY	
flexibility/adaptability	modify *only* if necessary
intent of activity	retain intent of activity
range of experiences	broaden range—risk taking?
	use New Games
	developmental
I. DESIGN SUPPORT SERVICES	
equipment/personnel services	provide adaptive equipment
	use support personnel

this section of the chapter and suggests some program strategies to address these variables.

Program examples.   The material that follows provides descriptions of two different and very successful projects that integrate disabled and nondisabled children and youth. Many other exciting and innovative programs that successfully bring people together are available to recreators.

PROJECT PLAE: Play and Learning in Adaptable Environments

ARTS AND ENVIRONMENT WORKSHOPS

Make a kite and paint it with your own personal design or logo. Learn to play the gamelan, a group of Indonesian musical instruments including giant gongs, drums and xylophones. Join the circus and be a tightrope walker, strongman, ringmaster or lion tamer. Search for buried treasure as an actress or actor in the full-fledged video production, "The Pirates of the Yard." Cook your own meals and converse with "visitors" from another planet.

These were some of the activities during Project PLAE's 1981 summer program, a series of week-long arts and environment workshops made available to children ages 6–16 in Berkeley, California, regardless of ability or disability.

Before the program got underway, there were skeptics. Few had tried to integrate disabled children into a program of activities usually reserved for nondisabled. Could severely disabled children participate without slowing others down? How would nondisabled children and their parents react? Could water, dirt, plants, trees—even fire—be used equally well by all children?

Fortunately, the optimism of Project PLAE's workshop leaders prevailed. They always found a way to involve even the most severely disabled. As Gina Moreland, co-leader of the Gardening and Cooking Workshop, said: "The kids were great. They really want to participate and giving recognition to that is vital. All children will let you know what they can and cannot do and what interests them."

Many parents were equally enthusiastic. "It's such a pleasure to see my daughter get dirty like any 'normal' kid. She's not fragile although she may look that way to strangers. It was even a pleasure to wash her dirty clothes knowing that she had a good time." Another parent felt very positive about having her two nondisabled children learn about disabilities firsthand to eliminate "any misconceptions or stereotypes they may have about special kids."

In fact, the children were probably the least aware of the unusual nature of the PLAE program. They played with each other, talked, laughed and learned together like any group of kids. There were enough heartwarming moments to convince any skeptic that integration can work.

Measuring Success

Many activities had an immediate impact back home. As one parent explained, "my daughter wasn't using her back-walker until she came home from playing circus and needed to practice her 'tightrope walking.' In fact, she was so fascinated by the whole circus thing she insisted we all go to the library one evening to get some circus books." Another parent told how her son wouldn't go to bed until he'd finished writing the script for the "Circus" performance the next day. A young girl in a wheelchair confided to her mother that she had a "boyfriend" at Project PLAE who helped her "do stuff." Another parent was ecstatic because for the first time in years she had found a program where both her children (one was disabled) could be enrolled. One child refused to eat breakfast the day of the gardening and cooking workshop so that she could cook her own at Project PLAE. To the pleasant surprise of one mentally retarded boy and his parents, he was cheerfully greeted on his first day at a regular school by two nondisabled playmates from the summer program.

Project PLAE began with one person making a phone call. A parent "discovered" the Environmental Yard one day while wheeling her severely disabled son around the neighborhood. She was immediately impressed by the calming effect the intimate landscape had on her son.

She called *Friends of the Yard* to ask if they could help set up a program so that more children with disabilities could use the Yard and play with the other neighborhood kids. *Friends of the Yard* were enthusiastic and willing to help. The network of connections began to grow.

More parents appeared on the scene—many of whom were frustrated after years of searching for integrated education and recreation programs of any type. The Berkeley Unified School District Office of Special Education offered meeting space and mailing services. A series of planning meetings were held. It was decided that community arts activities, coupled with the adaptable play area on the Environmental Yard, offered the greatest potential for involving children of all abilities.

Subsequent meetings were held on the Yard itself. Accessibility experts from the Center for Independent Living (CIL) in Berkeley looked at the site to identify potential accessibility problems. Picnics were held so kids could meet each other and begin exploring. Everyone learned from each other and what the Yard had to offer.

Community artists also began to appear on the scene. . . who knew other artists, who knew a friend . . . and so the network continued to grow. A group of musicians donated time for a fund raiser held at one parent's home. Many funding doors were knocked on, a few were opened. Eventually enough funds were collected to launch the summer program.

Place and Program: A Winning Combination

To make integration of disabled and nondisabled children possible, Project PLAE required an adaptable environment, a *physical place* of sufficient variety, that virtually any child could find something to explore. The Environmental Yard at Washington Elementary was just such a place.

The Yard provided the flexibility needed to create a *program of activities* with enough range and scope to effectively engage disabled and nondisabled simultaneously so that no child felt left out or unchallenged.

Arts and environment workshop became the backbone of the Project PLAE program. Professional artists and workshop leaders skilled in working with children were hired to run weeklong "theme" sessions. Leaders were given freedom to design and manage their own programs with assistance from other staff and interns.

Tuition was charged each child participant to cover basic costs and leader fees, which were based on the number of children attending.

For the most part, the ratio of able-bodied to disabled children was kept at two to one. Participants included children with cerebral palsy, orthopedic problems, Down's syndrome and other forms of retardation, brain damage and loss of hearing, one visually impaired and several with emotional and behavioral problems.

Two small grants, one from the East Bay Community Foundation (Oakland) and one from the Gannett Foundation (Berkeley), helped to defray initial start-up and publicity expenses and to provide a scholarship fund.

From *PLAE News*, Berkeley, California, no. 1, Spring 1982.

"COME FLY WITH US": A Mainstreamed Summer Day Camp Program

GIRL SCOUTS OF SANTA CLARA COUNTY, CALIFORNIA

"Come Fly With Us" is a day camp especially designed to mainstream girls into a regular day camp program. The fourth annual camp was held in June 1983 at Vasona Park, Los Gatos, California.

CAMPERS: Two one-week sessions were held with 144 campers in attendance. There were 67 girls with varying disabilities and 77 nondisabled girls. Thirty-two campers were non-Scouts.

STAFF: The volunteer staff consisted of 30 counselors, 7 support staff (director, co-director, registered nurse, registrar, and craft director), and 38 CREW girls (aides); 25 high school-age counselors (10 non-Scouts and 15 Senior Scouts); 12 adults (2 non-Scouts and 10 Scout Adults); 38 junior high-age counselors (5 non-Scouts and 33 Cadettes).

PROGRAM:

The camp program included all the standard Girl Scout Day Camp activities including cookouts, crafts, hikes, songs, skits, and games. This year we had an "Around the World" theme and "visited" a different country each day with crafts, food, posters, and dress appropriate for that country, ending the week with a Mexican Fiesta. We also had a ride on a miniature railroad, a visit from the local fire department, and a magic show by "Candy the Clown." The girls were placed in unit groupings and planned most of their daily schedule of activities with staff guidance.

RECRUITMENT:
(CAMPER)

The regular Girl Scout Day Camp folder was sent to all local troops and special flyers were sent to agencies and special schools that serve disabled children.

(STAFF)

Training information flyers were sent to Senior Girl Scout troops and all local high schools and colleges to recruit camp counselors.

TRAINING:

All counselors were required to take 40 hours of training relating to mainstreaming as well as day-camp program, or have the equivalent experience. As part of the training, all first-time counselors were required to help plan and staff a Play Day for disabled children, co-sponsored by the local Parks and Recreation Department.

TRANSPORTATION:

Thirty-eight girls with disabilities were transported by vans daily from all parts of the Council. Two local, specially equipped transportation companies were obtained to transport the girls.

COMMUNITY:

The community gave the program excellent support. Local businesses donated either camp supplies and time or gave significant discounts on the purchase of camp supplies. Local newspapers and television have given us excellent media coverage.

FINANCING:

The "Come Fly With Us" program is completely planned and staffed by volunteers; therefore, our camper fee of $15.00 per week, per girl, covered all the costs of the camp program. Donations for transportation expenses were received from the foundation—Corporation Summer Youth Project, Lockheed Bucks-of-the-Month-Club, and several local businesses and organizations. In addition, contributions were received from individuals.

EVALUATIONS: The main objective of the camp is to create a normal day camp setting where girls without disabilities and girls with varying disabilities could gain knowledge and understanding of each other as individuals by working and playing together. The camp was evaluated by campers, camp staff, parents, and community visitors. The evaluations were positive in both the aspect of camp program and the effectiveness of the mainstreaming process.

EXCERPTS FROM
EVALUATIONS   From a nondisabled camper: "This is the best camp I have ever attended. I liked everything except our burned pizza."

From a parent of a nondisabled camper: "I feel it was a great experience for my daughter. She has developed an understanding of what it means to have a disability and will feel more relaxed and comfortable with any disabled person she meets in the future."

From a parent of a disabled camper: "Thank you for the *very special* week at 'Come Fly With Us.' The week was an extremely happy experience and we appreciate all the time given by the Scouts to this project."

From a staff member: "I'm really glad I decided to work at camp this year. I hope this camp is around for my future daughters. P.S. See you next year!"

From a social worker who sent five girls to camp: "I am amazed at the significant positive changes in these girls after only one short stay at this camp. There is definitely an improvement in their attitudes about themselves and others. The total acceptance of everyone as an individual is a remarkable achievement by your camp staff."

From a flyer distributed by the Girl Scouts of Santa Clara County, California, October 1983.

SUMMARY

This chapter identified and discussed strategies for enhancing an individual's leisure expression and social interaction. The reader was given guidelines for designing programs and services that will lead to independent and interdependent leisure behavior of consumers.

The first section emphasized the major components or processes of leisure education: self-awareness; decision making; leisure-skill development; resource awareness and utilization; and social interaction. Through this discussion, the importance of leisure education as a major part of service delivery became evident.

The last section of the chapter addressed social interaction and social integration as focuses of therapeutic recreation and leisure services. Several factors critical to successful integration efforts were identified, and suggestions were offered for implementation strategies.

The chapter was intended to assist the reader in recognizing the learning processes that take place within leisure environments, and it suggested ways to maximize the positive effects of these processes.

DISCUSSION QUESTIONS

12-1. How did Mundy and Odum define leisure education? Define leisure education in your own words.

12-2. Discuss the relationship between leisure education and perceived competence.

12-3. Discuss the contribution of leisure education to the process of normalization (refer again to Chapter 9 if you need to refresh your understanding of this concept).

12-4. Five areas in which leisure education can make a significant contribution were presented in this chapter: self-awareness; decision making; leisure-skill development; resource awareness; and social skill development. What is the relationship of each of these areas to leisure independence? How are these areas developed through leisure education?

12-5. Several techniques to enhance leisure skills were presented. For each of these techniques, briefly define what is meant by the term, and describe how the technique can be used to enhance leisure skills.

transfer of benefits
activity analysis and modification
task analysis
developmental programming

12-6. What are some ways in which social skills can be enhanced?

12-7. What are some general guidelines for modifying activities?

12-8. The section addressing social integration and interaction relates particularly well to Phase III of the Humanistic Mainstreaming Continuum (Chapter 9). You may want to review these two sections together.

Several factors were identified (using a systems approach) that can contribute to the success of social interaction, particularly between persons who are disabled and those who are not. Describe the role of each.

physical environment
social environment
program structure/purpose
personal readiness
parent readiness
terminology
program content
staff attitude

CASE STUDY I

Work in groups of four to five people. Each group should review the case study presented at the opening of the chapter and then continue with the following directions:

1. You are the therapeutic recreation staff of this municipal therapeutic recreation department program.

   Decide who comprises the population being served by this social program, and briefly describe their overall behavioral characteristics.

   State the intended outcomes of this particular social development program; that is, what should participants be able to do (what social behaviors will they demonstrate) at the completion of the program?

   Develop an outline of the first 1-½-hour session of the 12-session program; specify what activities you will present, and what strategies you would use to teach these activities (keep in mind what one of the desired outcomes is).

   Select one of the activities you have chosen to present, and analyze and consider the modifications that might be necessary in order for the participants to participate successfully in this activity; use Table 12–3 as a guide.

2. After you have completed the above plan, present it to the rest of the class. If time permits, teach the activity, using the strategies you have identified and any modifications you believe to be necessary.

CASE STUDY II

In groups of five to six, students will select a role to simulate in making decisions about starting a socially integrated program. Select from among the following roles:

therapeutic recreator from United Cerebral Palsy Association
therapeutic recreator from a municipal recreation department
community recreator from a municipal recreation department

parent of disabled teenager

teacher of mainstreamed class (class has both able-bodied and disabled students in it)

As a group, you are interested in developing a program that brings together able-bodied and disabled teens in a fun-filled and attractive experience. Explore the following questions:

1. What should be the focus of such a program? Consider the type of program that would be of interest to this age group.
2. How will you attract both disabled and able-bodied teens to this program? How will you advertise? What kind of language will be used?
3. What kinds of skills or attitudes should participants in this program possess before entering the program? How can you be sure that participants will have these prerequisite skills?
4. How much information should participants be given about the nature of the program before it begins?
5. How can you ensure that all participants attain new skills and find maximum satisfaction through this program?
6. What will be the role of the therapeutic and community recreators in this program? Will additional training be needed by some staff members?

Consider the variables affecting the success of integrated programs discussed in the last half of this chapter. Also refer to the program examples for assistance in thinking through your program.

NOTES

[1] Jean Mundy and Linda Odum, *Leisure Education: Theory and Practice* (New York: John Wiley & Sons, 1979), p. 2.

[2] Jesse Dixon, "Recreation, the Disabled and the Search for Competence," *California Parks and Recreation*, Oct./Nov., 1981, pp. 14–15.

[3] Richard Page, Bill Holland, Mary Ellen Rand, Barbara C. Gartin, and Dian Aguar Dowling, "Assertiveness Training with the Disabled: A Pilot Study," *Journal of Rehabilitation*, April-June, 1981, pp. 52–55.

[4] Robert M. W. Travers, *Essentials of Learning*, 4th ed., (New York: Macmillan Publishing Co., 1977), pp. 385–418.

[5] Peggy Hutchison, "Maximizing Transfer Benefits of Special Programs," *Journal of Leisurability*, 2 (1975), 2–8.

[6] Carol Ann Peterson and Scout Lee Gunn, *Therapeutic Recreation Program Design: Principles and Procedures*, 2nd ed. (Englewood Cliffs, N.J.: Prentice-Hall, 1984), pp. 182–197.

[7] Target Access, *Closing the Gap: An Inservice Training Manual for Mainstreaming Recreation and Leisure Services*, San Jose State University (Oklahoma State University: National Clearinghouse of Rehabilitation Training Material, 1983), pp. 163–164.

[8] Paul Wehman, *Helping the Mentally-Retarded Acquire Play Skills: A Behavioral Approach* (Springfield, Ill.: Chas. C Thomas, 1977).

[9] Peggy Hutchison and John Lord, *Recreation Integration* (Ottawa, Ontario: Leisurability Publications, Inc., 1979), pp. 58–61.

[10] P. Wehman and J. Marchant, "Improving Free Play Skills of Severely Retarded Children," *American Journal of Occupational Therapy*, Vol. 32 No. 2 (1978), 100–104.

[11]Philip S. Strain, ed., *Social Development of Exceptional Children* (Rockville, Md: Aspen Systems Corp., 1982), p. v.

[12]S.L. Foster and W. L. Ritchey, "Issues in the Assessment of Social Competence in Children, *Journal of Applied Behavior Analysis,* 12 (1979), 626.

[13]Steven Asher and Angela Taylor, "Social Outcomes of Mainstreaming: Sociometric Assessment and Beyond, in Philip S. Strain, *Exceptional Children,* p. 14.

[14]Ibid., p. 23.

[15]Ibid., p. 23–24.

[16]Ibid., p. 24.

[17]Ibid.

[18]Hyman Hops, "Behavioral Assessment of Exceptional Children's Social Development," in Phillip S. Strain, *Exceptional Children,* p. 32.

[19]Richard P. Schutz, R. Timm Vogelsburg, and Frank R. Rusch, "A Behavioral Approach to Integrating Individuals into the Community," in *Integration of Developmentally Disabled Individuals into the Community,* eds. Angela R. Novak and Laird W. Heal (Baltimore: Paul H. Brookes Publishers, 1980), p. 108.

[20]Frank M. Gresham, "Misguided Mainstreaming: The Case for Social Skill Training with Handicapped Children," *Exceptional Children,* Vol. 48, No. 5 (February 1982), 422–433.

[21]Elliot Avedon, *Therapeutic Recreation Service: An Applied Behavioral Science Approach* (Englewood Cliffs, N.J.: Prentice-Hall, 1974), pp. 163–171.

[22]Phyllis Coyne, "Developing Social-Sexual Skills in the Developmentally Disabled Adult: A Recreation and Social Approach," *Journal of Leisurability,* Vol. 71, No. 3 (July 1980), p. 70.

[23]David J. Stang and Rick Crandall, "Familiarity and Liking," in T.M. Steinfatt, ed., *Readings in Human Communication* (Indianapolis: Bobbs-Merrill, 1977), p. 284.

[24]Ibid., p. 285.

[25]Ibid., p. 283.

[26]Robert C. Ziller and Richard Behringer, "Motivational and Perceptual Effects in Orientation Toward a Newcomer," *Journal of Social Psychology,* 66 (1965), 79.

[27]Gerald M. Philips and Eugene C. Erickson, "Entry into the Group," *Interpersonal Dynamics in the Small Group* (New York: Random House, 1970), p. 52.

[28]Monroe Berkowitz, Jeffrey Rubin, and John D. Worral, "Economic Concerns of Handicapped Persons," *White House Conference on Handicapped Individuals: Awareness Papers,* 1977, p. 220.

[29]William and Susan Stainback, "A Review of Research on Interactions Between Severely Handicapped and Nonhandicapped Students," *Journal of the Association for Severely Handicapped* (TASH), Vol. 6, No. 3 (Fall 1981), 23–29.

[30]S. McHale and R. J. Simeonson, "Effects of Interaction on Nonhandicapped Children's Attitudes Toward Autistic Children," *American Journal of Mental Deficiency,* 85 (1980), 18–24.

[31]Stainback, "Review of Research," p. 27.

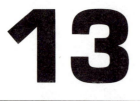

ENVIRONMENTAL INTERVENTION

As an organizer I start from where the world is, as it is, not as I would like it to be. That we accept the world as it is does not in any sense weaken our desire to change it into what we believe it should be—it is necessary to begin where the world is if we are going to change it to what we think it should be. That means working in the system.[1]

INTRODUCTION

The above words, written by Saul Alinsky, a noted community organizer, provide us with valuable insight and a foundation for our discussion of environmental intervention. Alinsky's simple truth is one that we must constantly remember and apply when implementing change strategies in our communities. One does not have to look very far to find ideologies, policies, or discriminating practices that have hindered the growth and development of individuals with disabilities. Alinsky advises us that bringing about change necessitates working within systems. Community acceptance and equal opportunities for people with disabilities will most likely occur in an environment where people do not feel attacked, put down, or alienated by therapeutic recreation specialists. When specialists understand a community's depth of knowledge about the needs of disabled people, they can then involve people in the change process who might otherwise be excluded.

We are responsible for working together to understand issues and concerns; to eradicate barriers to community involvement; and to design innovative strategies for solving problems. In order for these positive actions to become characteristics of future services, two factors that can account for change need to be recognized. First, there is a tendency in many social institutions to overemphasize the power of bureaucracy and to ignore the extent to which human choice can change the course of events.[2] Second, there is a tendency to adopt a static, rather than a dynamic, view of society.[3] Contemporary American society seems to emphasize social processes as continuous and made by people. According to Irving Tallman:

> Process and change are linked to man's capacity to learn and, by learning, to either adapt to or modify his environment. Social change results from constant interaction and feedback, which allows actors to assess the effects of their actions in terms of their goals.[4]

The recreation and leisure profession is viewed as a social institution in our society. According to Hertzler, the functional essence and the basic element of social institutions are that they are "systems of required, concerted, cooperative, and reciprocal practices or activities whereby the people concerned satisfy their individual and social needs."[5]

As a social institution, recreation and leisure service delivery systems are instruments through which social change is brought about. This complex concept of social change can be applied specifically to leisure services offered to individuals with disabilities; the direct application of this concept is the ecological perspective. Recreation professionals who operate within this ecological model can blend social action and community education to alter organizational structures, policies, and attitudes that place limitations on individuals with disabilities.

This chapter introduces both the concept and the process of change. Change and the rehabilitation process will also be explored in terms of their impact on the delivery of therapeutic recreation and leisure services. The barriers to equal access to services will be identified. Finally, this chapter will present a model for environmental intervention.

SOCIAL CHANGE

From the perspective of an individual, an organization, or a social system, nothing in life seems more certain than change. Change is inherent in human existence, an everyday aspect of social life. Within the next decade we will experience many opportunities for constructive change and immense progress as we encounter societal, organizational, and individual concerns and issues. These changes, at whatever pace, will affect every aspect of our lives. The challenge that confronts an individual, an organization, or a social system is to find a "promise of clear answers to basic concerns."[6]

Gray and Greben, writing about "Future Perspectives," clearly describe the impact social change has on the recreation movement. The authors state:

> Failure of the recreation and park movement to deal with change continually will inevitably lead to crisis. An adaptive mechanism that denies changes or denies the significance of change can only lead to failure. Adjustment to change requires flexibility and a short response time. Managing change requires a preferred vision of the future.[7]

Alvin Toffler vividly describes a concept of "future shock," which affects our communities, organizations, products, and even our expressions of concern, friendship, and love for one another.[8] Change in our society and in our lives can at times be a disruptive force that creates a fragmented existence, but the same reality of change can also become a plan of action to facilitate human development and reshape a fragmented society into an integrated whole. The need for a comprehensive plan of action is urgent as we plunge into the challenges of the next decade.

CHANGE AND THE REHABILITATION PROCESS

The rehabilitation process has traditionally involved the application of techniques and intervention strategies to change individuals. This process has often been conducted with the assumption that it is only the disabling condition that prevents the person from living and functioning in the mainstream of life. Roberta Nelson comments on another aspect of the rehabilitation process:

> The second half of the rehabilitation process must then be educating and training the community to accept people with differences and encourage them to live in the mainstream of life. Many obstacles still exist which prevent disabled people from living freely and fully. Just as there are barriers which prohibit disabled people from functioning in the community, so are there barriers which prevent the nondisabled from accepting the disabled as people with responsibilities and the right to live in the least restrictive environment as possible.[9]

Creating change within the community has been given a low priority by many members of the helping professions. We have failed to recognize that improving a person's ability to function independently does not always ensure community acceptance and support. An integrated body of knowledge regarding the process of planned change must be learned and applied by professionals. Resources for change need to be identified and shared to facilitate social, physical, and attitudinal changes within communities if people with disabilities are to be fully accepted and supported as viable citizens.

In the past decade our efforts have been directed at developing techniques and strategies to promote individual development, establish specialized services, and push for needed legislation. Looking back, the problem with this strategy is that we failed to work more closely with the general public in our communities. As a result, little has been accomplished in the area of community acceptance and support. One could dispute this argument by pointing out that more facilities are accessible, more services are available, and more disabled people are employed. However, we must recognize that the impetus for this "positive" response by society was the legislation that mandated these changes.

We all know that legislation alone cannot mandate attitudinal change. Fortunately, legislation has created certain physical changes in our environments. But faced with new issues and challenges as the nation's political outlook changes, we must work to prevent certain regulations and laws from being rescinded. We need the support of the general public. Unfortunately, in many communities public support is not readily available. In some instances we have not done an effective job of educating the community; professionals stand alone on some issues. We are now being accused of fighting only for our jobs at a time when organizations face severe budget cuts or changes in regulations and policies.

Members of the helping professions, and specifically therapeutic recreators, need to make a more serious commitment to develop additional strategies for community education and change. Obviously, our commitment to individuals with disabilities is a basic premise in the therapeutic recreation profession, but this belief in equal access and human development needs to be passed on to influential members of the general public if community acceptance and support are to become working realities.

BARRIERS TO EQUAL ACCESS

Research suggests that there are basically three types of change that are possible: evolutionary, accidental, and planned. The first two will not necessarily bring about the types of modifications important to creating community acceptance and support for people with disabilities. The third type, planned change, involves an organized, direct intervention in a human system to achieve specific goals. The ecological perspective to therapeutic recreation intervention is a direct application of planned change. Let us examine the barriers that hinder us from reaching our goal—creating community acceptance and support for people with disabilities.

Lack of Awareness

Many communities are not aware of the needs and barriers faced by people with disabilities. Nelson reminds us that "social change begins by communicating the need for change and then evolves through action and reaction."[10] Once the general public is more aware of the need for changing certain conditions and attitudes within a community, then there is value in having the public involved in the change process. Involving community members in change helps to educate society and serves to provide a smoother transition in eradicating barriers. Philip Mann states:

> The community must provide some sense of stability in the midst of processes of natural change, which means that it must to some degree be involved in planned processes of deliberate change that can maintain, and . . . enhance the quality of life of its members.[11]

Myths and Stereotypes

Another barrier to change relates to the myths and stereotypes of disabled people. Just as lack of knowledge can be a barrier so too can inaccurate information. The general public is plagued by misconceptions and fears—negative attitudes about the potential of people with disabilities, as we discovered in Chapter 5. Public attitudes need to be identified in any community change program. Creative problem-solving techniques may be implemented with success once myths are dispelled. George Albee sheds some optimistic light on the benefits of change. The author states:

> Frequently a revolution in scientific thinking occurs when some widely accepted premise, some "historical truth," is seen finally as inaccurate or incorrect. Our minds explore the crowded spaces created by the walls of fixed ideas until eventually we question why the walls are there at all. With the expanse of space that comes into view as the old conceptual walls are torn down, completely new kinds of explorations are possible. The simple step of abandoning an old, habitual pattern of thinking often leads to a whole new way of dealing with a problem.[12]

Learned Helplessness

The next barrier that we will examine is multidimensional. It is the theory of learned helplessness, which describes the type of behavior people may exhibit when they do not feel they have control over their lives. Helplessness often generates passivity and produces alienation. According to Sue and Zane, a relationship exists between the theory of learned helplessness and its application to the community. The authors observe:

> Where individuals in a particular community lack control, psychological well-being and the psychological sense of community may be diminished.[13]

Most people have experienced some changes in their contingent relationships. Traditional social institutions such as the family, church, and neighborhoods have increasingly lost their influence in our lives. Some of us may feel a sense of loss because at the same time that these institutions had influence over us, we also felt some degree of involvement and control over them. Institutions have comprised what we traditionally termed our community. Fortunately, the concept of community has evolved, and today it encompasses more than this traditional perspective.

What happens to disabled persons who feel a sense of helplessness in both their personal lives and in their communities? As suggested by Sue and Zane, this could result in diminished psychological well-being and in lack of a sense of community. One method of eradicating this barrier would be to plan a community education program that involves people with disabilities to help them regain some control and influence over their own environments.

Separate but Equal

The lack of exposure between disabled and nondisabled people is evident in almost every community. Segregation outweighs integration in our society. The range of segregation varies from large institutions, hospitals, specialized services, special schools, and other agencies. Thus, it is not surprising that we have not achieved positive social integration when the barrier of "separate but equal" is so prevalent in many communities.

This barrier can be easily justified because it relates so closely to several other barriers in community life. Researchers have examined the multidimensional nature of barriers and our need to be receptive to the multidimensional nature of their solutions. The authors of one such study state:

> Acceptance of difference comes through exposure. This means contact between handicapped and nonhandicapped people. Including handicapped individuals in community activities often provides opportunities for them to develop hobbies and interests with other community citizens. For example, unless a handicapped person is included in the YMCA, he might not have the chance to meet friends, who also like to watch league softball games. One contact often leads to another. Handicapped persons need the initial opportunities so that further relationships with people and involvement in the community can occur. Initial opportunities often depend upon the elimination of architectural barriers, provisions for public transportation, and citizen advocacy.[14]

Leadership and Power

A basic barrier to integration that is often overlooked relates to the concepts of leadership and power. Many influential members of our own communities are unaware of the changes that need to be made locally in order to create acceptance and support of disabled people. Many of them lack this awareness because service providers and consumers have failed to enlist them in their community awareness activities, in fund-raisers, or in special events.

Recreation professionals who act as agents of community change need power behind them if they hope to achieve the type of changes required. According to Nelson:

A change agent must recognize the social action processes as a series of stages from inception through legitimization, creating awareness, determining goals, mobilizing resources, action and evaluation. Understanding who the community leaders are, what their sphere of influence is, and at what point in the process they can be most potent is basic to creating change. A clear understanding of community power and leadership is required to ensure adequate consideration of community issues.[15]

Social, Political, and Cultural Elements

Social, political, and cultural elements characterize all communities, and these factors can be either assets or liabilities to the therapeutic recreator. When planning change strategies for our communities, it is important to note which of these elements could be potential barriers. Some of the community conditions that we should be aware of include the following:

1. Social policies
2. Program or department philosophies or ideologies
3. Cost control and cost-effectiveness issues/budget cutbacks
4. Service integration
5. Program planning and implementation; techniques, management
6. Organizational structures
7. Deinstitutionalization—community-based program trends
8. Social planning committees/advisory councils
9. Deprofessionalization—nonprofessionals, paraprofessionals
10. Political contingencies
11. Helping networks
12. Parent groups
13. Social characteristics of community residents
14. Behavioral patterns of target populations
15. Environmental conditions

Physical and Environmental Factors

Physical and environmental factors are additional barriers to community change and acceptance. These barriers are the most common types faced by people with disabilities and the ones most easily identified. Some of the physical or environmental factors in the community that hinder the independence of disabled people include the following:

Architectural Barriers (stairs, narrow doorways, high counters, phone booths, back door entrances, no consideration or accommodation for people with visual and/or hearing impairments)

Transportation (limited or lack of accessible public transportation)

Support Services (limited or lack of support services such as financial assistance, advocacy self-help groups, family support, leisure counseling, leisure education)

Resources (lack of resources for independence, independent living centers, skill-development programs, adaptive devices and equipment)
Community Recreation Services (lack of accessible and available community recreation programs and services for people with disabilities)

The barriers described above are the most common ones encountered in communities. Many of these barriers are also found in leisure-service agencies and departments within larger systems. Thus, the service provider has a responsibility at least to eradicate those barriers that hinder the leisure participation of individuals with disabilities. Failure to do so can have a negative impact not only on the disabled person but the community as a whole.

The *Assessment of Environmental Barriers to Leisure Experiences Instrument* (AEBLE) is designed to determine the most significant environmental barriers to recreation and leisure participation of orthopedically impaired children.[16] The developers of the instrument believe that environmental barriers are beyond the control of disabled children. The authors remark on the impact of these barriers:

> The presence of any or all of these factors tends to increase the dependency of the handicapped on others for satisfying their recreation activities. Skill development, enhanced self-worth, competence and socialization are all part of becoming a contributing member of society and fully enjoying leisure experiences. Identifying barriers to the development of these skills will allow the child and his or her support system to actively plan means of overcoming or circumventing these barriers and participating more actively in leisure.[17]

COMMUNITY DEVELOPMENT: CONCEPTUAL FOUNDATIONS AND PROCESSES

Because the concept of community development is complex, a framework will be presented by defining basic terms related to the concept and process.

These definitions are not to be interpreted as limiting or restrictive; they are a frame of reference for understanding and for future application. Definitions were selected from a review of the literature. It is the authors' intention to simplify the concept so that readers can focus their attention on the process of planned change.

Community

While community life has been disrupted, a new concept of community is suggested by the high degree of impermanence resulting from a nation of rootless people; one which is based on a greater degree of individual flexibility, vocational choice and selectivity, and leisure options within a highly mobile society. A new sense of community is emerging which transcends kinship ties, geography and social distance. There are no longer any natural geographical boundaries in the land that give a community identity. The traditional sense of community was largely rooted to the land and based on strong kinship affiliation. The new sense of community is predicated upon a wider community network, a common life style based on mutual compatibility and shared interests.[18]

Community Counseling

Community counseling is a multifaceted, human services approach. This approach combines experiential and environmental programs in order to help community members to live more effectively (and) prevent the problems most frequently faced by consumers.[19]

Community Development

Community development is the process by which people in an area, which they choose to think of as a community, go about analyzing a situation, determining its needs and unfulfilled opportunities, deciding what can and should be done to improve the situation and then move in the direction of achievement of the agreed upon goals and objectives. . . . Community development embraces both education and action, and the purpose of education is to prepare for intelligent action.[20]

Community Organization

Community organization is a method of intervention whereby individuals, groups, and organizations engage in planned action to influence social problems. It is concerned with the enrichment, development, and/or change of social institutions, and involves two major related processes: planning (that is, identifying problem areas, diagnosing causes, and formulating solutions) and organizing (that is, developing the constituencies and devising the strategies necessary to effect action).[21]

Community Psychology

Community psychology is, in part, an attempt to find other alternatives for dealing with deviance from societal-based norms. What is sought is an approach that avoids labeling differences as necessarily negative or as requiring social control. Community psychology viewed in this way is an attempt to support every person's right to be different without risk of suffering material and psychological sanctions.[22]

Social Action

Social action is employed by groups and organizations which seek to alter institutional policies or to make changes in the distribution of power.[23]

Social Policy

A social policy has been defined as a goal-oriented statement that identifies an existing societal problem or need and specifies a future condition in which the problem is reduced or eliminated. A statement of social policy generally leads to one or more sets of activities or programs that are designed to reduce or eliminate the problem. Social policies and their associated programs comprise statements of society's goals and the means designed to achieve these goals.[24]

Principles of the Community-Development Process

An effective community-development process is characterized by basic principles. These principles vary in their intensity, depending upon the model or approach used, the situation, and the leadership. These principles are significant and underlie the community-development process. Wileden has clearly and concisely stated some of these principles

1. The principle of need
2. The principle of agreed-upon goals
3. The principle of involvement
4. The principle of cooperation[25]

The process of community development is a movement toward the composite ideals of the many people who live in the community. The principles suggested herein, gleaned from scientific studies, from the experiences of many communities, and from the judgments of many community workers, are an attempt to provide an idealistic procedural frame of reference for a community inspired to work toward an ideal. They should be accepted in that spirit, followed where they prove helpful, modified where they appear faulty, and added to where they are inadequate.[26]

In addition to the above principles, Fessler has identified some basic guidelines that have proved to be helpful in bringing about change and in dealing with community problems. These guidelines can enhance the above principles and are included for our use.

First, attempts at planned change should be initiated at that level of community where people have a sufficient degree of primariness to make genuine interpersonal communication possible. In multicounty planning districts this means beginning with the separate county units, and in large metropolitan centers, the suburban and inner-city political jurisdictions.

Second, the more that community problems can be dealt with across institutional lines, free of the domination of any one institution, the greater will be the chances of breaking away from the limitations of the past and arriving at workable solutions that are in the interest of the total community.

Third, the more that concerned citizens outnumber bureaucrats in the decision-making process, the greater will be the possibility of putting the needs of the people above the survival of the bureaucracies.

And finally, to the extent that contemplated change will necessitate establishing new norms of thought and behavior for the community as a whole, it is essential that citizens representing organizations from all socioeconomic levels be included in the decision making.[27]

Resistance to Change

In any change effort there will be some resistance to change. The level or degree of resistance will depend on the people involved and the circumstances surrounding the change effort. Careful planning, organization, and sensitive leadership can reduce the negative feelings often associated with resistance to change. However, this resistance is a natural response shared by most people because change itself is typically seen as a disruptive force that threatens our security and life patterns.

Besides a general tendency to view change in a negative manner, there are many specific reasons why people may resist change. Thus, it is important to be aware of these before planning any change strategies. This preawareness will help us to plan more effectively, provide sensitive leadership, and allow us to be more prepared to deal with difficult situations.

1. *Negative attitudes toward change.* Beliefs and attitudes regarding change itself or the content of the change effort are negative. People who hold these beliefs or attitudes are not willing to examine how they have acquired these beliefs (cultural influences, parental influences, media, significant others) and change their attitude if the belief is based on inaccurate information. Perceptions are often distorted by cultural heritages.

2. *Poor Communication.* If people do not feel that they understand the nature of the change and/or do not feel it has been communicated effectively to them, they will not be supportive of the change. We all like to feel "a part of the action." Open and honest communication will usually help leaders gain respect and support for their ideas.

3. *Unclear purpose.* The purpose of any change effort needs to be clearly understood by all parties involved. An unclear purpose reflects poor planning and organization and results in a confused group with little or no unity and direction.

4. *Lack of involvement in planning.* Participation and involvement are two key principles of the community-development process. Without citizen involvement in the change effort there will be more resistance to change. The level of involvement depends on the situation, but this needs to be clearly understood and accepted by all involved.

5. *Norms and habits of the community ignored.* Every individual, organization, and community has developed behavioral norms and habits. Some of these are necessary for survival and organization. These norms and habits need to be acknowledged and respected. Remembering to start "where the world is" will ease transitions during change efforts.

6. *Fear of failure.* We often do not want to change or do something different because we are afraid of failing. We can learn from our mistakes, and this is often difficult. Change is not synonomous with failure. Encouragement and support will help us take some risks and learn from our experiences.

7. *Present situation seems satisfactory.* The need to change is not high when we feel that our present situation is satisfactory. We like to be comfortable, and when we know what is expected of us and can clearly define our parameters, change seems to serve no purpose. The desire to grow and develop becomes a personal decision.

8. *Cost for change is too high.* We are resistant to change when the cost for change seems too high and our reward for changing seems inadequate. Change may interfere with already established objectives—profits!

9. *Appeal for change is personal.* Change efforts that include a personal appeal for change are often resisted because they usually involve an emotional response. We often fail to trust our intuitive knowledge and experience or we lack an awareness regarding our capacity to use this dimension of ourselves.

LEADERSHIP AND COMMUNITY DEVELOPMENT

The process of community development is characterized by communication, planned strategies, organization, networks, and evaluation plans. These components require the skills of effective leaders. Niepoth has identified three leadership behavior characteristics, which are listed below:

> 1. Leaders develop congruence between their goals and group or individual goals.
> 2. Leaders make choices between the uses of persuasion and the uses of power.
> 3. Leaders consider their own personal characteristics and the characteristics of the group and the situation when selecting the approaches they will use.[28]

Leadership in this sense is not just dependent upon the qualities of the leader, but rather a complex interrelationship among many variables. McGregor has identified four major variables involved in leadership.

> 1. The characteristics of the leader.
> 2. The attitudes, needs, and other personal characteristics of the followers.
> 3. The characteristics of the organization, such as its purpose, its structure, the nature of the tasks to be performed.
> 4. The social, economic, and political milieu.[29]

There is no one leadership *style* for implementing planned change. However, basic leadership *skills* are needed to implement community-development action plans. These skills are organized into four major categories: (1) communication skills, (2) interpersonal-relationship skills, (3) self-awareness skills, and (4) organizational skills.

1. *Communication skills.* Communicating with individuals and groups is a major component of any community-development approach. The effective use of this skill will help to guide the planned change strategies and reduce a community's resistance to change.

2. *Interpersonal-relationship skills.* These skills are closely linked with communication but need to be considered as a separate entity. We have been discussing the concept of *process* throughout this chapter, and the significance of this concept cannot be overlooked. The relationships between people need to be developed and maintained. Socioemotional support can be facilitated by open-

ing up caring and responsible channels of communication. Trust and commitment are necessary to these types of relationships.

3. *Self-awareness skills.* The most important factor about individuals is how they feel about themselves. Much of the literature on leadership involves the acquisition of skills and knowledge in order to "lead" other individuals and groups. These skills are very important, but we must not overlook the importance of self-awareness. Brill provides some insight regarding the value of personal awareness.

> The worker who aspires to utilize himself in a disciplined and knowledgeable way in relationships with other people must have personal objectivity based on (1) awareness of himself and his own needs, (2) ability to deal with personality patterns within himself, and (3) resultant relative freedom from the limitations they may place on his ability to perceive with clarity and relate with honesty.[30]

4. *Organizational skills.* These skills (planning, organizing, evaluating, training) represent the basic skills required by most professionals who work closely with people.

Table 13–1 highlights specific leadership skills in each of the above categories. The student and professional are encouraged to add to this list based on their own personal experiences.

TABLE 13–1 Leadership Skills

COMMUNICATION SKILLS	INTERPERSONAL-RELATIONSHIP SKILLS
use verbal and nonverbal language	facilitate group process
use diverse forms of communication	understand and accept similarities and differences between people
practice perceptive and reflective listening	use appropriate mediation, negotiation, and advisement
apply objectivity	provide encouragement and support
send and receive clear messages	dynamiclly involve self in group process
give and receive objective feedback	develop congruence between goals and groups
integrate perception, culture, and context when interpreting communications	understand difference between content and process/task and relationship
use power and influence objectively	

SELF-AWARENESS SKILLS	ORGANIZATION SKILLS
demonstrate awareness of personal needs	conduct needs assessments
verbalize feelings	identify problems
demonstrate awareness of personality patterns	develop planned change strategies
develop ability to nurture self	develop evaluation plans
control self	advocate
demonstrate adaptive and flexible leadership styles	plan, implement, and evaluate training programs
	develop publicity
	identify and utilize resources
	identify supportive networks

ENVIRONMENTAL ECOSYSTEM
AND ACTION MODEL

The final section of this chapter presents an Environmental Ecosystem and Action Model. This model incorporates both the principles and processes of community development and change and the factors that have been discussed throughout this chapter.

Cooperation is a major characteristic of the model. Interacting in supportive and encouraging ways with people and our environment can be a determining factor in the success of change efforts. This type of social interaction can also help reduce the frustrations associated with change efforts by sharing the experience with a group of people committed to the same goals.

The cooperative approach to enhancing opportunities for disabled individuals is a difficult one to achieve. Elder comments on the barriers to this type of approach, barriers that need to be overcome if the approach is to be effective.

> The cooperative approach to serving persons with handicaps has been tried many times and many ways. Unfortunately, the success stories are few and the instances of "paper cooperation" too many. Many of these agreements are referred to as "warm fuzzies," which are simply promises to cooperate. Cooperation, however, has not necessarily resulted in implementation of more or better services. In many instances, the spirit of cooperation has not been supplemented with the concepts and procedures necessary to overcome the many governmental, organizational, and functional barriers which characterize all levels of bureaucracy.[31]

This model is designed to help both professionals and consumers examine their communities and environments, and it provides a structure to enhance a community and to direct positive social interaction.

> People have unique strengths and weaknesses that enable them to cope better in certain environments than in others. Consequently, we long for the best fit between persons and environments in general, not just the fit between a particular person and the best environment. This means that sometimes environments have to be changed to create meaningful and appropriate roles and ways of interacting.[32]

Creating community acceptance and support through the application of this model is its basic goal. The specific structure and function of the model will be described and illustrated. For now, let us examine the purpose of this approach. Nelson suggests that action groups are responsible for implementing community education and developmental programs. The author explains the purposes of this process:

> The purposes of a community education and development program are threefold. The first responsibility is to communicate the special needs and the po-

tential of disabled people, the existence of services for disabled people so that those who need the services may avail themselves of them, the need for services not yet available, the need for changing conditions which are handicapping to disabled people, the need for support, philosophical, volunteer, and financial. The second responsibility is to design the most effective way to create an atmosphere favorable to maximize the normalized living of disabled people in the community. The third responsibility of the program is to generate the needed philosophical, volunteer, and financial support to bring about the necessary changes.[33]

The first of three illustrations depicting the model shows the Environmental Ecosystem (see Fig. 13–1). The illustration displays the factors surrounding an action group that is charged with the responsibility of carrying out planned change strategies. These factors are forces that cannot be ignored but must be understood and accepted as natural parts of any system. They are the forces that can either guide or hinder the goals and objectives of environmental intervention.

In addition to these factors, there are four interrelated elements that

FIGURE 13-1 Environmental Ecosystem

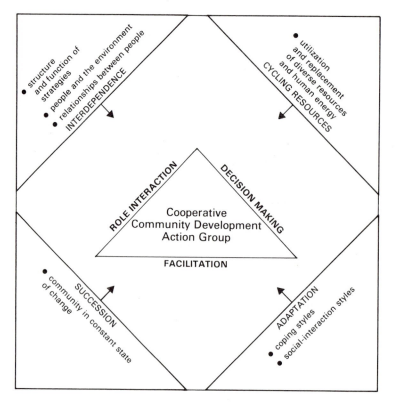

are constantly present during the change process: (1) interdependence, (2) cycling resources, (3) adaptation, and (4) succession. These elements are included in this model because they are what distinguish an ecological model from other community-development models.[34] This type of model views change as evolutionary and dynamic. Our communities are in a constant state of change, which is considered a *natural* state. Thus, these four elements are incorporated into this model as an integral part of its structure and function.

Our second illustration isolates the Cooperative Community Development Action Group. The four elements just discussed are part of the structure and function of the group itself. Three other components of the structure and function of the action group include: *role interaction, decision making,* and *facilitation* (refer again to Fig. 13-1). These three components are functions of a group process and serve to maintain group cohesiveness and progress toward agreed-upon goals. Figure 13-2 illustrates the group structure.

The last illustration of the model (see Fig. 13-3) presents the Community Development Training-Action Model. This part of the ecosystem is the same graphic structure as the Cooperative Community Development Action Group. This is significant in that the triangle is considered the strongest structure. The base of the model (assessment) provides the foundation. Once again, the four elements of an ecological model (interdependence, cycling resources, adaptation, succession) are present to provide consistency and sup-

FIGURE 13-2   Cooperative Community Development Action Group

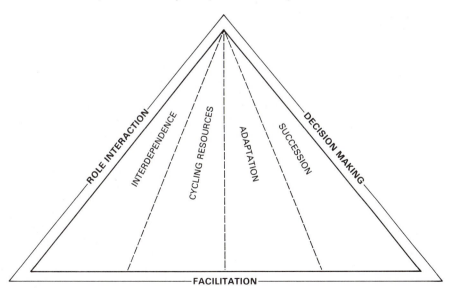

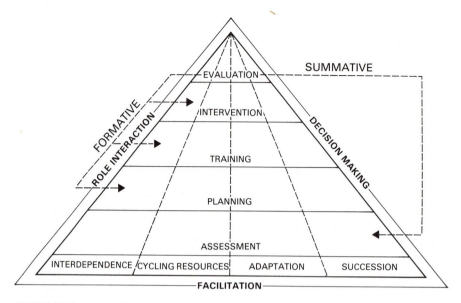

FIGURE 13-3 Community Development Training-Action Model

port. The functions of group process also surround the model to provide group cohesiveness.

The model itself shows the five actions of community development: (1) assessment, (2) planning, (3) training, (4) intervention, and (5) evaluation. (See Table 13–2, which describes the content and processes of each step of the model.)

TABLE 13-2 Community-Development Training—Action Model

ACTION	CONTENT	PROCESS
ASSESSMENT:	Community needs; community problems; barriers to equal access; existing services; resources; power structure; consumers; parents; professionals	Conduct surveys; hold community meetings; search directories; write letters to newspaper editors; hold public hearings; conduct interviews; review policy guidelines; establish advisory committees; establish cooperative interagency contacts; consult information and referral centers; contact media; consult self-help and parent groups; contact parent groups; contact service groups; contact voluntary action centers

TABLE 13-2   [*Cont.*]

ACTION	CONTENT	PROCESS
PLANNING:	Establish cooperative community action group; review assessment information; determine structure/function/roles of group; determine methods of communication; select group facilitation; describe problem; list possible solutions; set goals and objectives; determine planned change strategies; resources	Brainstorming meetings; interaction method for effective meetings; team building; nominal group process techniques; giving feedback, support; summarizing; conducting advisory meetings; clarification; probing and questioning; paraphrasing; active listening and reflection; analysis; decision making by consensus
TRAINING:	Assess training needs (based on skills needed to carry on planned action strategies); determine process and content for most effective learning; identify oral presentation skills; determine learning environment; determine training schedule	Andragogy (Adult Learning Process); identify and select trainers; conduct training program; evaluate effectiveness of training
INTERVENTION:	Rights and needs of disabled individuals; adaptive devices; community education; architectural barriers; community services; enhance integration; policies and procedures; power structure; resources	Information dissemination; community awareness/education events; develop partnerships between disabled and nondisabled people; mass media campaigns; interagency cooperation; disability awareness activities; skill-development programs; presentations; workshops; training; involve administrators in leisure programs; organize councils of disabled people; leisure education/leisure counseling; advocacy; environmental barrier modification; compile and publish a community services directory; involve parents as educators; involve consumers in education/awareness events; review policies and ideologies and make recommendations to appropriate boards and commissions.

(*continued*)

TABLE13-2   [*Cont.*]

ACTION	CONTENT	PROCESS
EVALUATION:	Purpose of evaluation; criteria; audience of evaluation; how evaluation data will be used; resources and constraints	Select appropriate evaluation methods (triangulated); formative evaluation; summative evaluation; conduct evaluation; analyze data; report data; reassess needs

SUMMARY

Environmental intervention is a process involving many factors. Process and change are essential to our ability to learn and grow. The factors and principles of environmental intervention are interactive and dynamic. Thus, those who seek to effect change in their communities must constantly be aware of the dynamic quality of change inherent both in human interactions and in the interaction between individuals and their environment.

This chapter presented a model for developing change strategies in our communities in order to bring about environments and organizations that seek to accept and include individuals with disabilities as viable members. This model is an ecosystem and encompasses the factors that impact upon intervention plans. Taking these factors into consideration helps therapeutic recreation specialists design realistic plans of action to include all members of a community who might lend support.

DISCUSSION QUESTIONS

13-1. What are some of the barriers that may hinder the community's acceptance of individuals with disabilities?

13-2. What principles are important to the process of community development?

13-3. Why do people and organizations often resist change?

13-4. What leadership skills are important for professionals to possess when implementing community-development action plans?

CASE STUDY

A city Park and Recreation Department has recently hired you to develop a recreation program for children with disabilities. The city has a positive relationship with the school district. An initial assessment was completed for the city by the volunteer recreation commission, where the need for this service was identified. You have begun your position as a program coordinator and soon discover the following community conditions:

a. the community center building is not physically accessible;
b. there is no accessible public transportation;
c. the recreation staff is resistant to working with disabled people, and they don't feel adequately trained;
d. the director of the department does not understand the purpose of therapeutic recreation services.

Applying the Community Development Training–Action Model, how would you solve these problems? Suggestions for starting: How would you assign priorities to the problems? What people or organizations may be supportive to you and the new program?

NOTES

[1]Saul Alinsky, *Rules for Radicals* (New York: Vintage Books, 1971), p. xix.

[2]Irving Tallman, *Passion, Action and Politics: A Perspective on Social Problems and Social Problem Solving* (San Francisco: W. H. Freeman & Company Publishers, 1976), p. 252.

[3]Ibid., p. 253.

[4]Ibid.

[5]J.O. Hertzler, *American Social Institutions* (Boston: Allyn & Bacon, 1961), p. 84.

[6]"Challenges of the 1980s," *U.S. News and World Report*, October 15, 1979, pp. 45–55.

[7]David Gray and Seymour Greben, "Future Perspectives," *California Parks and Recreation*, June/July 1974, 11–22.

[8]Alvin Toffler, *Future Shock* (New York: Bantam Books, 1970).

[9]Roberta Nelson, *Creating Community Acceptance for Handicapped People* (Springfield, Ill.: Chas. C Thomas, 1978), p. 9.

[10]Ibid., p. 33.

[11]Philip A. Mann, *Community Psychology* (New York: Macmillan, 1978), p. 321.

[12]George Albee, "A Competency Model to Replace the Defect Model," in *Community Psychology: Theoretical and Empirical Approaches,* eds. Margaret Gibbs, Juliana Lachenmeyer, and Janet Sigal (New York: Gardner Press, 1980), p. 213.

[13]Stanley Sue and Nolan Zane, "Learned Helplessness Theory and Community Psychology," in *Community Psychology: Theoretical and Empirical Approaches,* p. 121.

[14]James Paul, Ann Turnbull, and William M. Cruickshank, *Mainstreaming: A Practical Guide* (New York: Syracuse University Press, 1977), p. 36.

[15]Nelson, *Creating Community Acceptance,* p. 179.

[16]Peter A. Witt, David M. Compton, Jim West, Ann Costilow and Melville J. Appell, *Manual for Utilization of the "Assessment of Environmental Barriers to Leisure Experiences" Instrument* (Denton, Tex.: North Texas State University, Division of Recreation and Leisure Studies, 1981).

[17]Ibid., p. 8.

[18]James F. Murphy and Dennis R. Howard, *Delivery of Community Leisure Services: An Holistic Approach* (Philadelphia: Lea & Febiger, 1977), p. 64.

[19]Judith Lewis and Michael Lewis, *Community Counseling: A Human Services Approach* (New York: John Wiley & Sons, 1977), p. 15.

[20]Arthur F. Wileden, *Community Development: The Dynamics of Planned Change* (Totowa, N.J.: The Bedminster Press, 1970), p. 80.

[21]George Brager and Harry Specht, *Community Organizing* (New York: Columbia University Press, 1973), pp. 27–28.

[22]Julian Rappaport, *Community Psychology: Values, Research and Action* (New York: Holt, Rinehart & Winston, 1977), p. 1.

[23]Brager and Specht, *Community Organizing*, p. 27.

[24]Lyle P. Wray, "Social, Political and Cultural Challenges to Behavioral Programs in the Community," in *Helping in the Community: Behavioral Applications*, ed. Gary Martin and J. Grayson Osborne (New York: Plenum Press, 1980), p. 355.

[25]Arthur F. Wileden, *Community Development: The Dynamics of Planned Change* (N.J.: The Bedminster Press, 1970), pp. 277–283.

[26]Ibid., p. 284.

[27]Donald R. Fessler, *Facilitating Community Change* (San Diego, Calif.: University Associates, 1976), pp. 12–13.

[28]E. William Niepoth, *Leisure Leadership: Working With People in Recreation and Park Settings* (Englewood Cliffs, N.J.: Prentice-Hall, 1983), pp. 130–135.

[29]Douglas McGregor, "An Analysis of Leadership", in *Leadership and Social Change*, eds. William R. Lassey and Richard R. Fernandez (San Diego, California: University Associates, 1976), pp. 18–19.

[30]Naomi I. Brill, *Working with People: The Helping Process* (New York: J.B. Lippincott, 1973), pp. 1–2.

[31]Jerry O. Elder, "Coordination of Service Delivery Systems," in *Planning for Services to Handicapped Persons*, eds. Phyllis R. Magrab and Jerry O. Elder (Baltimore, Md.: Paul H. Brookes Publishers, 1979), p. 196.

[32]Paul E. Stucky and J. R. Newbrough, "Mental Health of Mentally Retarded Persons: Social-Ecological Considerations," in *Living Environments for Developmentally Retarded Persons*, eds. H. Carl Haywood and J. R. Newbrough (Baltimore, Md.: University Park Press, 1981), p. 44.

[33]Nelson, *Creating Community Acceptance*, p. 42.

[34]Mann, *Community Psychology*, pp. 189–192.

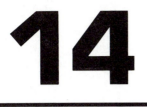

LOOKING TO THE FUTURE

A new civilization is emerging in our lives, and blind men everywhere are trying to suppress it. This new civilization brings with it new family styles, changed ways of working, loving and living; a new economy; new political conflicts; and beyond this, an altered consciousness as well. . . . The dawn of this new civilization is the single most explosive fact of our lifetime.[1]

INTRODUCTION

Throughout this text we have examined therapeutic recreation services in the context of the society in which we live. We have also commented throughout that this profession, as are all responsible and viable institutions, continues to change and mature, both from internal pressures and external forces.

As a student preparing to enter the field or as a professional already practicing, you no doubt can see the necessity for keeping abreast of societal trends. Shifts in attitudes, politics, and the economy; demographic changes; technological and communication advances—all are among those major factors impacting upon our profession.

Therapeutic recreation personnel are faced with tremendous challenges as we enter the last decade of this century. We are called upon to analyze our services against the backdrop of dramatic shifts in society.

We are going through a period now in which we are totally restructuring the United States. We are rebuilding the social, political and economic institutions to conform to the needs of a new economy and a new society.[2]

To remain viable requires vision; we will not survive if we make decisions based solely on "That's the way we've always done it." Our actions and practices will continue to challenge us to combine our theoretical knowledge, excellent technical skills, and a solid understanding of self with an understanding of what is happening in society. For those who would prefer cookbook-type answers to the challenges ahead we can only reiterate that we know of no foolproof answers. Ambiguity seems to be a reality of life—sometimes uncomfortable but always intriguing.

This chapter, then, offers no pat solutions for where our profession should go in the future. We can only raise some critical issues that are imminent and suggest ideas for your consideration. By being aware of these and other issues, together we can collaborate to discover meaningful solutions.

APPROACHES TO PREPARING FOR THE FUTURE

We can think about the future from several perspectives. Deciding upon a career is one example.

How did you select your career—or what steps are you going through now to make a decision?

1. You are following your parent's wishes. They have always wanted you to be in leisure services or therapeutic recreation. Or you are purposely going against your parent's wishes. Either way, your decision has something to do with your parents.
2. You are pursuing an old interest. Perhaps you were in a youth group or volunteered for some human-service activity. Or maybe you have always loved what recreation does for your own life. You want to continue this enjoyment into your future career.
3. You fell into it. You met another student in this major and became curious. Perhaps you talked to a friendly professor in this field who suggested you look into it. Or maybe you ended up in a leisure-studies classroom instead of a calculus classroom and decided this was more interesting.
4. You have strong ideals about what you think society "should" be like. You envisioned a better place or way to live and decided that by being a professional in this field, you could help achieve this dream.
5. Others. Certainly this list isn't exhaustive.

The ways in which we decide upon careers are similar to the ways in which people prepare for the future, period. The first two responses outlined above are based upon trying to fit our future into something we connect with the past. Our experiences and the messages we have been given by others play a predominant role. Thus, both the wisdom and folly of our past shape our future.

The third response cited above is a bit haphazard. Here there is very little planning—things just "sort of happened." This is known as "going with the flow" or listening to our intuition. We react to a set of circumstances.

The fourth response requires that we think of how we would like conditions to be. This is referred to as a "preferred future." The starting point is the future. We plan in reverse to determine how to arrive at that future point. We create our future.

You likely used more than one approach to decide upon a career path. All the approaches seem to be helpful to us in planning for the future. Certainly we can never escape our personal experience, regardless of how objective we try to be. And if we always plan in the context of the future, we may miss the opportunity of the moment. Yet if we have no vision of where we would like to go and how things might be better, our future will be circumscribed by unnecessary limitations.

With these approaches in mind, consider the following issues.

FUTURE ISSUES FACING THERAPEUTIC RECREATION NOW

In selecting the following issues (there are others as well), we consulted the writings of such futurists as Alvin Toffler, Buckminster Fuller, and John Naisbitt.[3] Futurists specialize in identifying current societal trends and forecasting future ones. In recent years, a few leisure researchers have used special forecasting methodologies to provide insight into the implications of these trends for the profession.[4]

From a Postindustrial to a Communications Society

Remember trying to imagine what it must have been like for people in an agrarian society to adjust to an industrial society during the Industrial Revolution? Yet here we are in the middle of the most dramatic societal changes since that time. We are currently experiencing the Technology and Communications Revolution—the movement away from a postindustrial society to what Alvin Toffler termed the *third wave.* Technology and access to information envelop us.

Technology in its broadest sense is the application of an organized body of knowledge to practical purposes.[5] As it relates to therapeutic recreation, that encompasses physical objects, such as wheelchairs and other adaptive devices, as well as processes, such as our delivery systems. The possible uses of technology to enable persons with disabilities to achieve goals related to a satisfying leisure lifestyle are limitless.

Technology has enabled individuals with spinal cord injuries to walk; the human voice has been simulated; the quality of life has been enhanced by the advent of less burdensome medical equipment; and home-bound individuals have found new connections with the outside world through computer networks.

Yet the costs and risks associated with technological development must also be recognized. For example, the futuristic book *Megatrends* provided evidence that people have a need to balance technology with some kind of human interaction, or "touch."[6] In other words, as high technology (technology associated with electronics, computerization, and so forth) expands, the need for "high touch" also dramatically expands.

Certainly this is a message to human-service providers. (Often the strongest arguments for our profession can be found in sources outside the field.) We are faced with a unique challenge to find a balance in the high tech–high touch dilemma. To ignore technology and to avoid participation in deciding its uses in the profession would be a waste of valuable resources for the recipients of our services. Conversely, to be consumed by technology would reduce our viability in providing the human interaction so fervently sought by others.

The importance of technology would certainly point to the need for professionals to be comfortable with its various forms and, in fact, to be technology-literate. It would seem that professional preparation programs must include basic computer literacy for all leisure-studies students.

Many questions exist; begin by considering these:

In what ways could technology be effectively used to assist persons with disabilities achieve personal goals related to leisure?

What kinds of therapeutic recreation/leisure services can we provide that will most likely respond to the need for "high touch"?

What roles should therapeutic recreators assume in the development of appropriate technology?

Demographic Changes

Reports in the daily newspapers as well as from futurists remind us that the demographic character of the country is undergoing vast changes.

Far from the concept of the "melting pot" is the ethnic and cultural diversity of our communities. The rapid growth in recent years of both the Spanish-speaking and Asian-American population has caused us to rethink our perspectives. And within every ethnic or cultural group, whether black, brown, yellow, or white, there is incredible diversity. By 1990, it is expected that Spanish-speaking Americans will be the nation's largest ethnic group.[7] And by 1992, it is predicted that California will become the first mainland state with a nonwhite majority. (Interesting, isn't it, that we do not even have appropriate terms to describe this situation? "Nonwhite" is still based on a predominant concept of "white".)

Of course our country is aging as well. A decline in the birth rate combined with improved medical technology has resulted in a growing percentage of Americans living past the age of 65. Older Americans, as a population, have become very articulate about their needs; they have developed a powerful base from which to effect economic, political, and social changes.

Certainly these major demographic trends will have a tremendous impact on service delivery. How should we respond? In what ways should our services, our roles, our interventions, our thinking be changed? How can professionals prepare themselves to be effective service providers under these new conditions?

Standardization

Most futurists agree that our society cannot be governed by any one set of standards. Social structures, the economy, and all types of services—education, health, leisure—will look different from one region to another because of the great diversity that exists throughout the nation. Futurists believe that the "standards" approach advocated in earlier decades will have little place in our new society.

Our professional organizations have worked diligently to identify standards of practice in therapeutic recreation. Indeed, standardization has been identified as one mark of our profession. These standards help upgrade the provision of services by setting a minimal level of services that must be provided in any quality program.

Does this represent a conflict between the direction of our profession and the direction that society is headed? How can we reconcile this apparent discrepancy? To what point should national standards be accepted and at what point should local needs determine local service delivery? Given that we are concerned about the *quality* and adequate quantity of services, how do we ensure both in our own communities?

Recall that many therapeutic recreation professionals worked with allied professionals and consumers to get federal legislation passed that mandated the levels and types of services provided. How can we continue to work toward this end?

Specialization

Leisure services, like most other professions, have developed several specialties within the field (therapeutic, commercial, employee, outdoor recreation). According to Alvin Toffler, specialization in the work place served a particular function during the industrial era; namely, to accelerate production (mass production), thus saving time and energy. Further, diversity among jobs represented a needed balance to the homogeneity that evolved in language, leisure, and lifestyle.[8]

Toffler states:

> . . . specialization was accompanied by a rising tide of professionalization. Whenever the opportunity arose for some group of specialists to monopolize esoteric knowledge and keep newcomers out of their field, professions emerged . . . the market intervened between a knowledge-holder and a client, dividing them sharply into producer and consumer.[9]

Toffler and others suggest that specialization was a product of a fragmented, segmented, industrial, and postindustrial-based society.[10] Its usefulness, however, is limited in a "new-order" society where access to information is a way of life and where people are entering more collaborative relationships and self-help orientations.

In many leisure service/therapeutic recreation settings, the limitations of specialties have already been addressed. Therapeutic and other recreation personnel are *networking* to share resources and provide services more effectively. Networking, or connecting with others who have similar needs, interests, and goals, is also evident among public and private agencies.

Other professional activities within therapeutic recreation are contributing to the further specialization of the field. Efforts to license therapeutic recreators, for example, are a reflection of the medical/legal professional model that has interest in its own self-protection. Of course, most therapeutic recreation practitioners have entered the fight on behalf of licensure to save therapeutic recreation services from extinction in medical/rehabilitation settings, and to articulate the importance of leisure in life. It is believed that licensure will also help secure third-party reimbursement for services.

Yet a conflict is evident: Will licensing or other activities that contribute to specialization (and standardization) help us in being more viable as service providers, or will those activities give us a false sense of security? Will we slip into oblivion as we become entangled in the folds of a useless, protective cloak? Finally, will our acceptance by the existing medical and political structure benefit consumers?

The Self-Help Movement

For decades, people relied on institutions to assist them in meeting needs related to education, health, employment, and recreation. This dependency on external help is rapidly giving way to independence and mutual support. The rise in self-help is evident in every facet of life; see Table 14–1.

The growing self-help perspective in recreation and leisure perhaps became most apparent during the taxpayers revolt of the late 1970s. Although not directed solely at leisure services, the voters' message was to reduce both

TABLE 14-1   Institutional Versus Self-Help Approach

INSTITUTIONAL APPROACH		SELF-HELP APPROACH
ILLNESS:		PREVENTION:
doctor diagnosis and treatment	*Health*	shifts in eating, fitness patterns
medicine and surgery for healing		reduction in smoking
little personal involvement or responsibility		lifestyle patterns changing
		mental/attitudinal healing
		high degree of personal involvement and responsibility
schools and their personnel are responsible for majority of teaching	*Education*	parents assume greater responsibility for teaching
officials make decisions		parents play a greater role in decision making
public sector is large and is a primary employer	*Careers*	private sector attracts more people
large organizations		small organizations
management of long-established enterprises		venture projects, entrepreneurial activities
career counseling		career exploration with peers
supermarkets	*Food*	community gardens
		food coops
		farmer's markets
		preserving own food
use of programs provided for specific needs and interests	*Recreation and Leisure*	people with mutual interests form own programs
staff plans facility uses		neighborhood swim and tiny-tot programs
public departments maintain facilities		special interest programs such as whitewater-river rafting trips
		people request use of public facilities for their own planned events
		neighborhood provides upkeep of facilities

the costs and the extent of publicly supported services. Mistrust of the public sector loomed large in the minds of many people.

As we discussed earlier in this text, the disabled community has actively developed self-help groups to assist members in developing independence and control in their lives. Therapeutic recreators have been in a unique position; as "friendly" professionals, they often work closely to support self-help activities.

Considering the tremendous transition that has been made from reliance on institutional systems and professionals to reliance on self, professionals in our field should consider what new roles we might assume within this context. Will our importance as facilitators and enablers increase? Do we need to rethink how we presently provide services? To what degree are participants or their advocates involved in decisions related to services? How can we increase our viability?

New Directions in Health

Several factors have helped elevate health care to a prominent national concern, not only today but over the next several decades:

1. Health care costs have skyrocketed in recent years. Medical/hospital fees are beyond the ability of many people to pay, creating problems of access to the system. Low-income people are severely affected by these costs. Even insurance premiums have been so costly that they are difficult to pay out-of-pocket.
2. The growth of America's older population has put pressure on the health care system. Advocates are fighting for equality in access to this system through new legislation, including nationalization of health care.

From cure to wellness.   The trends toward self-help, individualization, and a new consciousness about personal responsibility have contributed to the "wellness" concept. Rather than relying on the medical profession to treat an illness, people are taking action to remain well. Fitness, nutrition, smoking, drinking, leisure behaviors, and related behavioral patterns are being evaluated in favor of healthier lifestyles.

Concerned about higher costs of traditional health benefits (insurance coverage premiums, for example) and lowered productivity by employees from days lost to illness, employers are examining health care alternatives. Many private corporations and public-sector employers have opted to include a wellness component as part of their health care benefit packages. Typically, these services include exercise and fitness programs, nutritional support, recreational activities, and specialized services (antismoking classes, weight loss, stress management).

The competencies of professionals prepared in therapeutic recreation can make a significant contribution to these services. With the focus on leisure lifestyle satisfaction, these professionals can collaborate with employee recreation personnel to individualize services. Through the use of individual assessment, goal setting, activity planning, and evaluation, programs can be implemented to help individual employees (and their families, as appropriate) to attain healthier leisure patterns that contribute to their total wellness lifestyle. Therapeutic recreation personnel can use their expertise in leisure education, mental health, and related areas to contribute significantly in programming areas.

Given that therapeutic recreation is partially based on the concept of wellness (prevention), the link with employee (sometimes called *industrial*) recreation seems obvious. And given the growing awareness of employers to health care costs, this would appear to be a growth area within the professional market.

However, before we make the leap into this sector, we should address these questions:

> What kinds of knowledge and skills would therapeutic recreators need to possess in order to work effectively in corporations (beyond the competencies they would be expected to possess in more traditional settings)?
>
> How could therapeutic recreators articulate to corporations what they have to offer?
>
> How can therapeutic recreators and employee recreation personnel collaborate effectively?

The holistic health movement.   Closely related to the concept of wellness is that of holistic health. This movement was discussed extensively in relationship to rehabilitation (see Chapter 11), but deserves consideration in a broader context.

This approach to health is more than a trend or a fad. It is an attitude, a way of looking at life, a perspective of the world that is an integral part of the perceiver. It requires a vision that supersedes intellectual thought and which incorporates intuition. It requires that one see connections among life's various parts, and it synthesizes seemingly isolated events into a unified whole. More than a professional concept, it is a personal belief and a way of living.

As such, not all therapeutic recreators will see the significance in the relationship between therapeutic recreation and holistic health beyond the intellectual connection. For many, the connection will be evident; for some, it will be the magic. For within this paradigm, the art and science of the profession are intimately integrated. The intuitive, creative, transcendental, spiritual self—the truly playful self—balances the rational, logical, physical, active being. By combining our professional skills with our personal vision, we can create environments and guide experiences that lead people into the new realms.

A few therapeutic recreation professionals have ventured into this new land. One such example is "Squnch," a magical journey created for children by Barbara Hanes-Morse, a therapeutic recreator in a residential treatment center for emotionally disturbed children.[11] Using imaginary creatures uncurling from their shells to explore worlds of purple velvet hills, lavender seas, "poet trees," and more, the "Squnch" stories guide children through their own experiences—their own barriers, pains, joys, and possibilities. These stories, which have been reproduced for distribution to the general public, are yet another affirmation of our potential contributions not only to health but also outside of traditional environments.

More questions are raised for your consideration:

How does a therapeutic recreator successfully articulate the holistic health perspective within a more traditional health care setting?

Given the demands of life, how does a therapeutic recreator—or any allied health or human-service professional—sustain a balance between the rational and the intuitive, between the creative and the mundane, between the spiritual and the physical domains in their own lives?

SOME CLOSING THOUGHTS

The questions raised about our profession are not ones easily answered. Yet they point to issues that must be acknowledged and addressed. Simply to jump on the professional train to go for a ride without asking its destination or without making sure it is even on the tracks may leave one stranded in the midst of nowhere. Involving oneself in the dynamic development of a field as exciting and challenging as this one, on the other hand, can be both personally and professionally rewarding. Simultaneously, critical thinking and questioning with follow-up action on the part of professionals is critical to the continuing evolution of therapeutic recreation.

DISCUSSION QUESTIONS

14-1. What are some ways to plan for the future, as outlined in this chapter? How do you typically plan for your own future?

14-2. This chapter identified a few of the major challenges that therapeutic recreation will face in the future. For each challenge, only a few main points were discussed. In small groups, select one issue to explore in more depth and present your findings to your class. Issues that could be selected include:

The use of technology in therapeutic recreation.
What effect will the changes in technology have on therapeutic recreation?
Should we support further standardization in our field?
Should we become more, or less, specialized?
Therapeutic recreation and the self-help movement.
The effect of changes in the health care system on therapeutic recreation.
Therapeutic recreation and the holistic health movement.
Other issues?

NOTES

[1]Alvin Toffler, *The Third Wave* (New York: Bantam Books, 1980), p. 9.

[2]Michael Annison, "Naisbitt Executive Delivers Moving Megatrends Message . . . ," *Dateline: NRPA*, Vol. VI, No. 10 (December 1983), p. 6.

[3]Toffler, *Third Wave*; Buckminster Fuller, *Critical Path* (New York: St. Martin's Press, 1981); John Naisbitt, *Megatrends: Ten Directions for Transforming Our Lives* (New York: Warner Books, 1982); Marilyn Ferguson, *The Aquarian Conspiracy* (Los Angeles: J. P. Tarcher, 1980).

[4]Karla Henderson and M. Deborah Bialeschki, "Public Urban Recreation in the Future," Madison, Wisconsin, Recreation Resource Center, 1982.

[5]*Technology and Handicapped People,* Office of Technology Assessment, Washington, D.C., May 1982, p. 51.

[6]Naisbitt, *Megatrends*, pp. 39–54.

[7]Ibid., p. 246.

[8]Toffler, *Third Wave*, pp. 49–51.

[9]Ibid., p. 50.

[10]John Lord, Peggy Hutchison, and Fred Van Derbeck, "Narrowing the Options: The Power of Professionalism in Daily Life and Leisure," in eds. Thomas Goodale and Peter Witt *Recreation and Leisure: Issues in An Era of Change* (State College, Penn.: Venture Publishing, 1980), pp. 228–245.

[11]Barbara Hanes-Morse, *Squnch*, "Magical and Motivational Program, Using Original Music," audiotapes produced by Chevron, U.S.A., Inc.

INDEX

introduction, 1–2
philosophical development, 163–69
professional development, 163–69
recreation model, 165–66
treatment model, 166
Therapeutic recreators:
change agents, 26, 276–77
attitudes, 36–37
characteristics, 27, 71
registration, 37
responsibility, 93, 117–18
role models, 83
service roles, 25–26, 34–37
Therapeutic recreation service:
activity model, 43
clinical or medical model, 19, 48
conceptual foundations, 4–8, 165
concerns (figure), 22
definition, 8–10
ecological model, 19–20
guidelines for working with disabled
people, 139–40
historical perspective, 144–63
age of consumerism, 154
agrarian society, 144–45
colonial American, 147–49
equal rights era, 155–56
folk era, 144
Greek and Roman era, 145–46
industrial era, 149–51
medieval period, 146–47
social reform period, 151–52
World War II, 152–53
professional roles, 190–91
social reform/community development model, 19, 48
therapeutic community/milieu therapy model, 20
therapeutic recreation service model
(figure), 57
transitional, 186–88
Third party reimbursement, 237–38
diagnostic related groups, 237
Transfer of benefits:
definition, 247–48
Transitional service, 186–87, 244–45

Veteran's Administration Hospital, 43

Well-being (see wellness; see health):
role of humor, 60–61
Wellness (see health):
intact strengths, 60

leisure, 61
personal control, 60
Wheelchair programs, 153
Witchtrials, 148

AUTHOR

Addams, Jane, 15
Alinsky, Saul, 274
Allport, Gordon W., 27

Bell, Alexander Graham, 151
Ball, Edith, 55
Bank-Mikkelson, 174
Barnett, Lynn, 53
Berryman, Doris, 56
Blatt, Burton, 117
Blocher, Donald, 27–28
Brill, Naomi, 17–18
Buchanan, Paul C., 29
Buscaglia, Leo, 105, 110

Compton, David, 35, 43
Cousins, Norman, 32
Czikszentmihalyi, Mihaly, 51

DeGrazia, Sebastian, 44
Dix, Dorothea, 150

Ellis, Gary, 206, 207 (table), 228

Fessler, Donald R., 37
Ferguson, Marilyn, 25
Fishbein, Martin, 82
Frye, Virginia, 56, 71

Gallaudet, Thomas, 150
Gardner, William, 120
Gray, David, 164, 276
Greben, Seymour, 276
Greenberg, Sheldon, 34
Gunn, Scout, 35, 56, 57 (figure), 221,
242

Howard, Dennis, 18–19 (table)
Howe, Samuel Gridley, 150
Hutchison, Peggy, 35, 179–81, 229,
247–48

Iso-Ahola, Seppo, 44, 45, 46, 227